THE
ULTIMATE
GUIDE TO
EMOTIONAL
HEALING
WITH
CRYSTALS & STONES

Understanding and Applying
Stone Energy to Achieve
Inner Harmony and Peace

UMA SILBEY

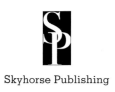

Skyhorse Publishing

Text and Photography Copyright © 2023 by Uma Silbey

Special thanks to Leah Francisco for modeling.

Skyhorse Publishing books may be purchased in bulk at special discounts for sales promotion, corporate gifts, fund-raising, or educational purposes. Special editions can also be created to specifications. For details, contact the Special Sales Department, Skyhorse Publishing, 307 West 36th Street, 11th Floor, New York, NY 10018 or info@skyhorsepublishing.com.

Skyhorse® and Skyhorse Publishing® are registered trademarks of Skyhorse Publishing, Inc.®, a Delaware corporation.

Visit our website at www.skyhorsepublishing.com.
Please follow our publisher Tony Lyons on Instagram at @tonyisuncertain

10 9 8 7 6 5 4 3 2 1

Library of Congress Cataloging-in-Publication Data is available on file.

Cover design by David Ter-Avanesyan
Cover photo credit: Uma Silbey

Print ISBN: 978-1-5107-7649-4
Ebook ISBN: 978-1-5107-7650-0

Printed in China

This book is dedicated to those medicine men and women, shamans, yogis, and meditation teachers as well as to my professors at UCLA and CIIS who passed their knowledge to me, believed in my potential, and encouraged me to share what I learned. Thank you for your faith in me.

TABLE OF CONTENTS

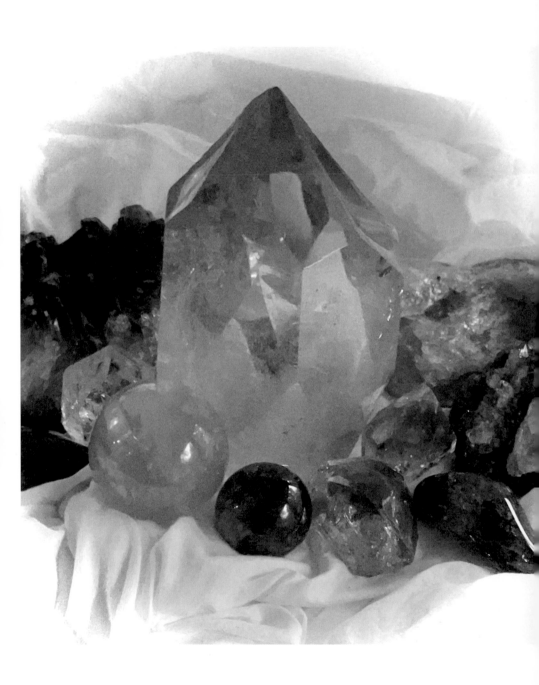

INTRODUCTION

Emotional Healing with Crystals & Stones
A Journey of Discovery

This book is designed to be instructional, thought-provoking, and inspirational. It is intended to bring you an opportunity to gain an extensive level of expertise so that you can examine and heal your own emotional pain as well as that of others. Rather than presenting you a mere list of stones and their properties, you will be offered much more: specific techniques and well-tested, effective methods to work with them so that you can become a masterfully effective emotional healer.

To start your emotional healing journey, a brief examination of how crystal healing works will be presented to you along with the importance of focused intention and a short discussion of the placebo effect. This first section will guide you to deeply examine and become familiar with the underlying basis that supports and empowers all forms of emotional and other forms of healing. Simple crystal techniques will be revealed to you that will help you achieve the "empty mind" and one pointed focus needed to perform this healing work.

The next section of this book will explore the transitory nature of emotions and their potential to be destructive to your sense of well-being. Emotional layering stemming from early childhood core wounding is explained with examples. Knowing the dynamics of emotional layering and core wounding, you can understand the difference between surface feelings and those deeper, more pervasive ones that support the superficial. Recognizing this, your healing can reach beyond the obvious outward emotions to those that are deeper. When these deeper levels of emotional pain are recognized and transformed to emotional peace, permanent emotional healing can occur. Clear examples will be presented of each type of typical emotional layering. Methods will be revealed to show you how to use your crystals to safely reveal each emotional layer and bring healing as it unfolds.

Along with emotional layering, typical destructive early childhood decisions that are consciously and unconsciously made based on those core wounds are examined. Since these self-destructive decisions are the ones that form the unconscious need for emotional layering to avoid facing emotional pain, it is important to reveal the original wound. When you can enable the healing of both surface and core emotional pain, your emotional healings will be powerful and lasting.

After exploring core wounding, you will be presented with a list of the most important emotional healing crystals and stones, as well as a general description of their use in emotional healing. These are divided between heart stones or crystals, protection crystals, stones and crystals for communication, insight, and trust. These will allow you to build your initial "emotional healing crystal kit." Alongside these crucial crystals, additional emotional healing crystals and stones are presented for their "fine tuning" effects.

After learning about the best emotional healing crystals to have in your emotional healing kit, you will be presented with the specific emotional healing techniques (with pictures) that you can do with them. First, you will be shown some general emotional healing techniques. Following this, specific crystal healing techniques for thirteen commonly recurring emotional upsets will be provided. Pictures of stones, crystals, and healing patterns accompany each one of these treatment explanations. After that, eleven of the most typical core wounds that you will encounter in your emotional healing work will be presented. Accompanying this description of the most typical core wounds is a list of the most typical defensive patterns you may find when trying to heal core wounding.

Practicing the impactful and thought-provoking techniques presented here will enable you to become a master emotional healer with your crystals and stones. Hopefully, you will also have a chance to experience an expanded level of being that will bring you happiness and inner peace, so that as you heal others, you will also be healed.

> ### AS YOU HEAL OTHERS,
> ### YOU WILL ALSO BE HEALED.

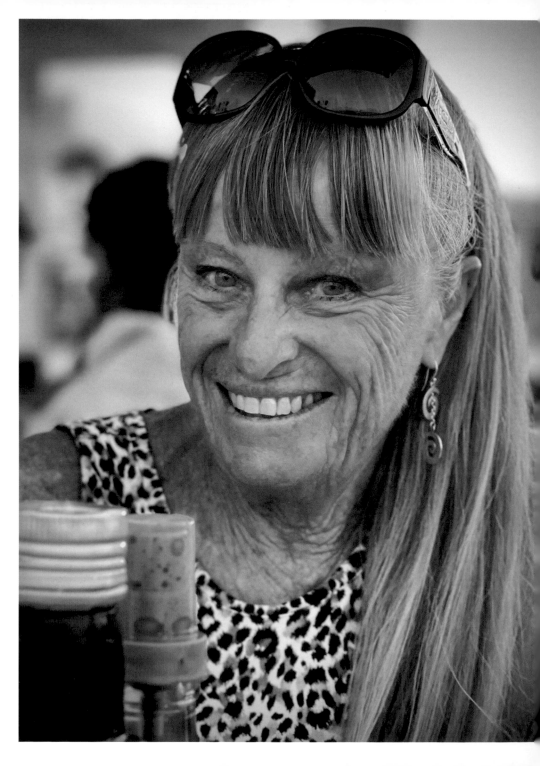

ABOUT THE AUTHOR

I have been actively working with crystal and stone healing for more than fifty years. As long as I can remember, I have felt the energy of stones. When I started making gemstone jewelry in the seventies, I usually matched specific stones with my clients to help balance their energy. At the time, I didn't know it was "energy balancing" or that it was unusual to be able to "feel" the stone's energy, much less match it with the energy of anyone else. I just recognized that certain stones seemed to be good to use with certain people. It helped form the basis of my early jewelry work.

I have also been doing yoga and various forms of meditation since the seventies. Among other things, this has helped me be very cognizant of subtle energy and states of being well beyond the physical. I am very aware of kundalini energy, the chakra system, and other subtle energy pathways in the body and how they connect with emotions and thought. These yoga and meditation practices also further enhanced my sensitivity to the subtle energies connected with the crystals and stones. The stones "speak" to me quite clearly. For years, then, I have combined this awareness of the physical, mental, and emotional subtle energy patterns with that of the crystals and stones.

I encountered my first quartz crystal about fifty years ago and was immediately aware of its associated energy. When concentrating on this first crystal, in my "mind's eye" I immediately "saw" exactly how to use them. It was as if I had had lifetimes of experience earlier. All I had to do was focus on a problem and its crystal solution presented itself to me. This ability to "hear" the crystal is what underlies successful crystal healing work.

This is not to say I have not also been trained. I studied crystal and stonework with several Native American Medicine men and women and various shamans and yogis through the years. Interestingly, though, as soon as I learned a new technique, it was as if I had always known it.

Besides the metaphysical training, I have also been well trained in more traditional psychology and psychological therapy and counseling work, both at the University of California at Los Angeles (UCLA) and the California Institute of Integral Studies (CIIS). I have worked with gestalt therapy, couples and family therapy, Jungian therapy, integral therapy, music therapy, group therapy, and psychodynamics. I have also worked with psychobiology and research psychology. I have hours of counseling experience in a more traditional office setting as well as the work I do on an everyday basis. I also have a master's degree in counseling psychology as well as a professional counseling psychology certification.

This book, then, combines my psychology background and my metaphysical background with my years of work with crystals and stones. It also builds on the information contained in my prior books, from the first crystal book I wrote in the early eighties to the present.

I offer you the benefit of my all my years of training and experience in this writing of this book. It is my hope that you be successful in all your emotional healing endeavors with the crystal and stones and that their "voices" may resound loudly and clearly within your heart and inner awareness.

SECTION ONE
PREPARATION

Before You Begin a Meditation

Whenever you perform one of the meditations or any of the other techniques, unless you are instructed otherwise, begin by sitting upright with your spine straight, either on a straight backed chair or in lotus or half lotus yoga pose. Rest your hands faceup in your lap, your arms and legs should be uncrossed, and your feet should rest on the ground or floor. Face straight ahead with your chin dropped about an inch so that it feels as if the back of your neck gently stretches upward. If you don't sit upright, lie down on your back with your head straight, arms at your sides, your palms upward, and your legs uncrossed with your feet next to each other.

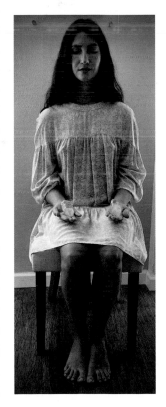

Begin by calming your mind, centering, balancing, and grounding yourself. To center yourself, begin with long, deep, easy breaths and imagine that they flow in and out of your heart center in the middle of your chest. After a minute or whenever you feel calm and a sense of being gathered into your center, ground yourself. To do this, feel your connection with the earth by imagining long, earthen-colored roots extending from the bottoms of your feet deep into the earth. As you do this, first imagine breathing inward through your heart center in the middle of your chest. Then extend the roots downward with each out-breath. Do this for a minute. Then balance your grounding by continuing to imagine your in-breath flowing into your heart center, and then with each out-breath, imagine the top-center of your head opening and a beam of clear, golden light streaming upward into the heavens. Do this for another minute. Finally, bring your attention back to your heart center and imagine your breath again flowing in and out of it. Once you are done, remain focused on your heart center as you do your crystal emotional healing while being grounded and balanced.

Storing and Clearing Your Emotional Healing Crystals

Crystals not only amplify and transmit energy, but they also become naturally programmed, (take in and store energy) from anything with which they come into contact, whether that is thought, sound, speech, feelings, physical bodies, or active use. This, in turn, will tend to affect you or the other person as you use these crystals, or even if you have them in the environment with you. Unless you intend to use this programming, it is important to be sure you clear any of this stored energy before using your crystals again. This is especially true if you have used them for a prior emotional healing session in which you have worked with negativity or emotional trauma.

You should clear your emotional healing crystals immediately after each healing session. Then wrap them in a natural fiber cloth or put them away in a pouch. It is recommended to use a dark fabric for the best shielding. You may, however, decide to use a color with which you want to charge your healing crystals for its healing effect. You may, for example, want to use a purple cloth for its positive influence on the upper wisdom energy centers. Likewise, you may want to use a green

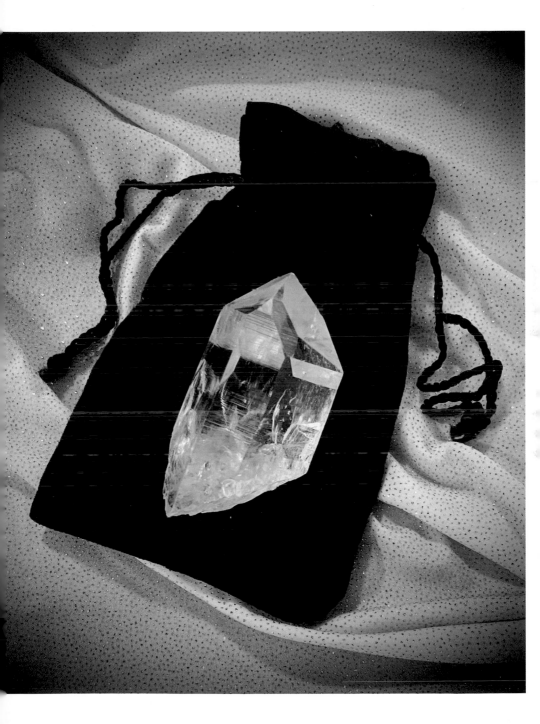

or pink cloth for its stimulating and opening effect on the heart center. One drawback to this, of course, is that you are then limited to this color in your next session until you clear the energy from the crystal. Be cognizant of your color combinations, also. Neither black nor white will interfere with a crystal's energy. However, if you combine a different color cloth than your emotional healing crystal, you will have influenced your crystal with two colors, the color of the cloth and the color of the crystal. A blue crystal wrapped in a yellow cloth is generally not good, for example, as the sun of the cloth may interfere with the blue crystal's energy, negating its "blue" effects.

There are many ways to clear a crystal. One of the easiest and most effective ways is to smudge them by blowing smoke from various herbs, cedar, or sage over the crystals with the intention that they be clear. Do this until they seem clear. You will have a clear sense when this has occurred if you are paying close attention. It feels somewhat like how you feel when you straighten a crooked picture on a wall. There is a sense of "whew" or "aha" that is unmistakable. Using the smudging technique has many benefits, among them the ability to smudge many crystals at once, the entire room or environment, yourself, and the other you are working with. You should clear or smudge the environment in which you are doing your emotional healing crystal work, the other person, and yourself before you get started and after you are finished. The smudging method will never damage a crystal as salt does (or some of the other clearing methods that are sometimes used).

Crystal Preparation

Unless there are other instructions how to use your crystals during any of the emotional healings, use these. Place a single terminated, clear quartz crystal in each hand as they rest upward-facing in your lap. The crystals will work more effectively if they are clear rather than cloudy or dull. They should be at least three inches long and an inch wide. Point the

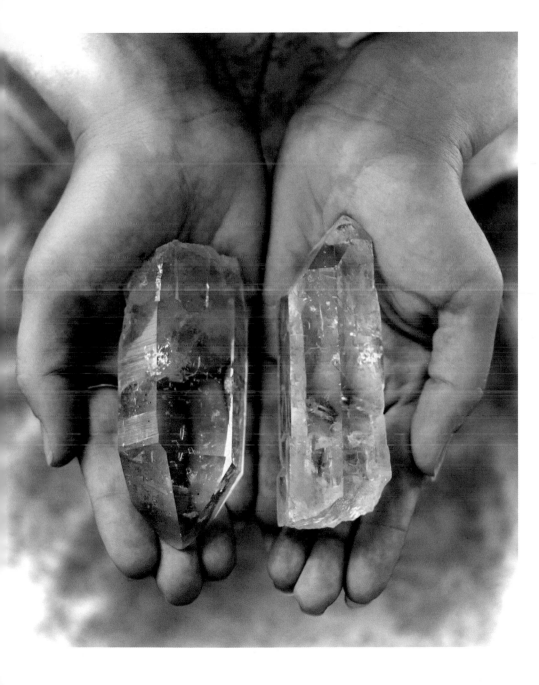

crystal that is in your left hand upward toward your arm. This is the receptive crystal. It will amplify and help receive any communications or realizations as they occur during your emotional healing. Point the crystal in your right hand outward, its tip extending toward your fingertips. This is the expressive crystal, its energy flowing outward to amplify the work you are doing and enhancing any communications so they are clear for you and the others you may be working with.

You may also use large Herkimer diamond crystals, one in each upward-facing hand. Herkimer diamonds are double terminated, very bright, and generally the most powerful of all the quartz crystals. Because they are double terminated, each crystal both sends and receives energy. Because of their strong energy, they will vitalize your entire body and help open your higher energy centers to increase your awareness and subtle "hearing."

CRYSTALS WITH POINTS ON ONE END ARE CALLED **SINGLE TERMINATED.**
CRYSTALS WITH POINTS ON BOTH ENDS ARE CALLED **DOUBLE TERMINATED.**

To further enhance your emotional healing, wear or place a rose quartz, pink tourmaline, pink calcite, pink rhodonite, or pink rhodochrosite over your heart center. A 24-inch chain will generally place a crystal over any person's heart center unless they have a large body or neck. Then you will probably need to use a 26-, 27-, or even a 30-inch chain.

A green crystal also works well to stimulate the heart center. Generally, you should use green for actual physical heart healing, or when nurturing is particularly needed. Pink crystals, though, are typically used more for emotional work, softening, and gently revealing the deeper emotions of the heart. If you do use a green crystal, a lighter, softer, more gentle green color is generally recommended for emotional healing work. Try using a green calcite, light green jade or serpentine jade, or a light green fluorite.

These crystals, of course, are not the only crystals to use during an emotional healing session. You will learn others later in this book. These, however, will get you started.

Creating a Safe Space

Since deep emotional turmoil is a symptom of early core wounding and the unconscious attempts to defend against the resulting feelings, any time you use your crystals to do any kind of emotional healing to remove

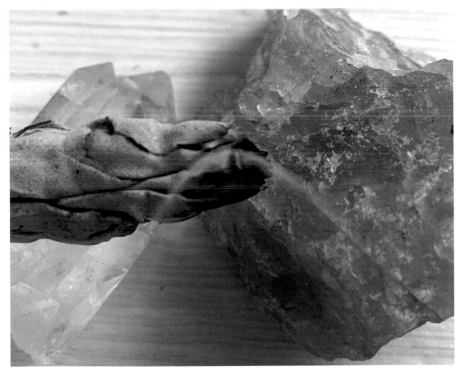

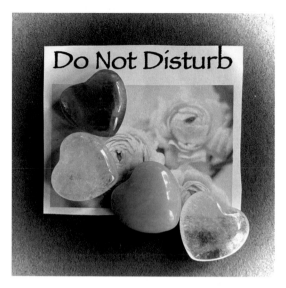

these painful defensive feelings can be quite scary. It is of utmost importance, then, to create a space or environment in which the person being healed feels safe enough to reveal and release their emotional defenses.

To create an environment that is supportive of emotional expression, you must make sure that no one or nothing will intrude or interrupt you. Turn off your phone, for example, and make sure your pets stay out of the room. You may want to put up a sign on the door of the room letting people know not to knock or come in. If you are creating an office or special room in which you will do your crystal emotional healing work, perhaps paint the walls a peaceful color like light green, mauve, or light violet. Rid the room of any clutter except for two comfortable places to sit facing each other at a distance that feels nonthreatening yet interactive. Plants create a good energy to have in the room. You can also put up one or two pictures with peaceful topics. Quiet water like an expansive, calm ocean or lake helps generate feelings of peace, as do single roses, lilies, lotus designs, or mandalas. Again, don't clutter your room with too many pictures. There should be a sense of space as well as peace.

You can use your crystals to help create a sense of a safe space. You can place rose quartz, amethyst, and other healing crystals in the room in which the emotional healing will occur. You can create a healing grid of energizing crystals around the room, charging them with healing visualizations and connecting their energy to surround yourself and the one being emotionally healed. Crystal balls are excellent to use for this as the round shape creates a soft and peaceful presence even though they are powerful.

> ## ONLY WHEN SOMEONE FEELS SAFE
> ## CAN THEY REVEAL THEIR DEEPER SELF.

The Power of Nonjudgmental and Complete Listening

During any emotional healing session, you must be able to *thoroughly listen to the other* without interrupting or correcting them. To let them know you are listening, you can ask them if you have understood them, saying something like, "I hear you saying this." Then repeat what they have said to you and ask if you have heard correctly. In these ways, the other person can feel completely heard in a way that perhaps they may never have been heard before. The power of this type of active and complete listening to another is often vastly underrated. Being heard without judgment can be emotionally healing just in itself.

Completely listening to another means that you must listen without judging them in any way. They must feel completely accepted no matter what they say or what they reveal. In listening this way, don't correct anything about the feelings they are revealing or anything about them as a person. Let them know with your complete, nonjudgmental listening that they are okay just as they are, that they are not deficient in any way, that they matter to you, that nothing is wrong with them no matter what they reveal to you. This way they can feel free to cry, rage, or let out any other "negative" feeling and you will not flee, and you will still stay emotionally open and available to them. In other words, you are a safe "container" for their deepest feelings. No matter what they say, they will not drive you away. This not only lets people release the repressed feelings, but it also models that it is safe to be self-expressive. The more accepting of them you are, the more they can be accepting of themselves in their entirety. The more accepting of themselves they can be, the more they can be accepting of and in true relationship with others.

Being nonjudgmental doesn't mean you can't discriminate. You can accept an emotional communication in its entirety and still see how it doesn't serve them. You can accept an emotional expression and still work to change it.

Nonjudgmental listening does not mean that you must be a depository for abuse. If the other is striking out at you with their words, attempting to hurt you as they feel hurt, it is okay to stop them and let them know that you are feeling abused then model more appropriate emotional expression by reframing what they say without any blame. For example, if they are calling you names, let them know that when you hear these words you feel angry and that you suspect, perhaps, that this is how they feel about themselves. Ask them to take a breath, and then ask them to investigate their feelings to see if this is so.

NONJUDGMENTAL AND COMPLETE LISTENING IS EMOTIONALLY HEALING JUST IN ITSELF.

The Ultimate Guide to Emotional Healing with Crystals & Stones

SECTION TWO
HOW CRYSTAL HEALING WORKS

At heart, all that exists is essentially space, a limitless state before awareness and beingness. This state cannot be mentally understood or explained, as it has no form nor beginning or end. As manifestation comes into being from this formless state, it expresses itself as vibration. All that is manifested, from the physical to thoughts and emotions, is formed as a particular vibrational pattern. These vibrational patterns are what we alter to make the positive changes that we do in all crystal healing, including our work with emotional healing.

Since everything in existence is a manifestation of a vibrational pattern at its heart, when that pattern is changed, there is a corresponding change in the outward manifestation. This is true of the physical manifestations, but also emotional, mental, psychic, and spiritual manifestations. Each physical object vibrates differently from the other. Each feeling vibrates with a different rate, each thought is expressed with a different vibrational pattern, and so on. So, if you change anything in manifestation, you change its vibrational pattern. The more focused and clear minded you can be, the more your sensitivities can expand past the physical into the subtle realms. Then you can feel or sense these vibrational patterns.

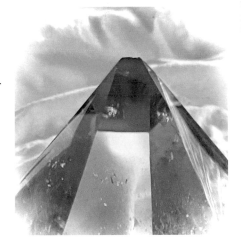

In the case of emotional healing, to change the emotion, you change the vibrational pattern associated with a negative or painful emotion or emotional pattern to one that corresponds and supports more positive emotions. One way to work to alleviate sadness, for example, is to use your crystals to help shift its slower, heavier-feeling vibration to the quicker, lighter vibration associated with joyfulness. You can also use skillful communication and 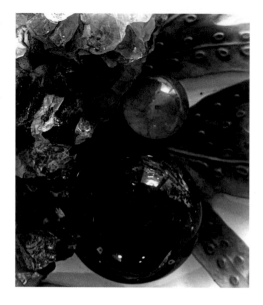 focused intention to shift the vibrational patterns of difficult emotions to those that are more pleasant. When you use your crystals to do emotional healing work, you use them in certain ways, coupled with skillful communication, to assist this vibrational change.

You can use your crystals to make these emotional vibrational changes in many ways:

1. You can physically manipulate your crystals and stones to activate this vibrational change. You can use your crystals or stones to raise subtle energy, lower it, cut through it, extract it, or transmit it to change the original vibrational pattern to one that corresponds to positive changes in the outward emotion.
2. You can use your crystals to help you be more concentrated and clear-minded so that you become more aware of these subtle energy patterns and how they need changing.

3. You can use them to extend your own awareness so that you can more easily "read" someone's emotional state, both its more obvious outward appearance and that which is buried beneath layers of emotional protection. You can use your stones to increase your awareness so that you "hear" or "see" the depths and nuances beneath a more outward emotional expression and know how to change it and what to change it to.

You are not limited to actively using your crystal to raise, lower, remove, replace, or otherwise alter the vibrational patterns in another. You can do this for yourself also, using the same techniques. It is easier, though, to heal someone else rather than yourself because you can be more objective with another person. When working to heal yourself, it is easy to be blinded by your own subjectivity and be swayed off course by your own thoughts, desires, beliefs, and feelings about yourself or your condition. In other words, you can think you are one way or another and entirely miss the way you really are. You may think, for example, that you are generally happy and use those thoughts or beliefs to hide your own depression.

Using Your Crystals to Change Vibration

Follow these steps to use your crystals to change vibration.

1. Center, ground, balance yourself and quiet your mind.
2. Have the other person stand or sit opposite you with their hands facing upward as if receiving the energetic change that you will induce. Before beginning, have them breathe with long, deep, breaths in and out of their heart center. This will calm their mind, bring them to the present, and open their receptivity.
3. Hold a clear quartz charging crystal in your left hand with its tip pointing upward toward your arm in receptive position. Hold

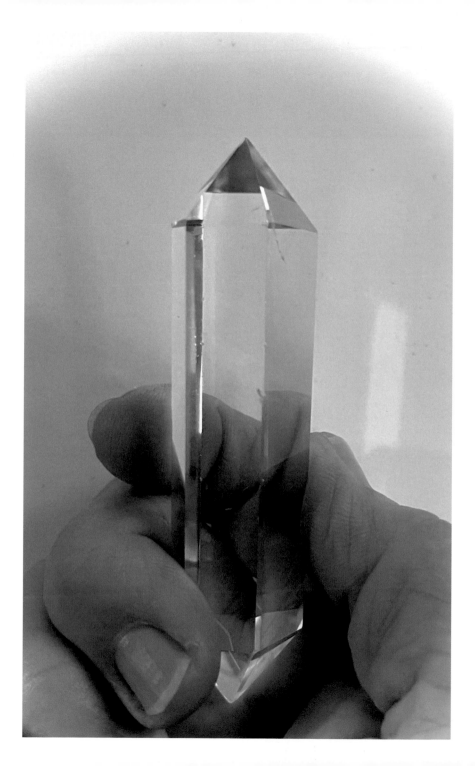

another same-sized clear quartz crystal in your right hand with its tip pointing outward toward the other person.

4. Focus on your third eye to increase your intuition and awareness of subtle energy.

5. Intuit, sense, or "see" the other's energetic state that represents their emotional imbalance. With the intention of correcting the imbalanced energetic state with one of balance, point the crystal in your right hand toward the person or the location in their body where the imbalance seems to be.

6. Use this crystal to energetically rebalance their energy by "pulling out" the negative energy while visualizing replacing it with positive energy. You can also send in energy where the other's energy seems to be depleted. You can sweep your crystal upward from their feet to their head to raise their overall energy rate if it seems depressed or low. Alternatively, use your crystal to sweep from their head to their feet to lower their energy if it feels frantic or overactive.

7. Continue doing this until you sense, "see," or feel that you have achieved your goal.

8. You can also visualize sending in color when needed. You can draw out the gray of depression where you find it in the body and send in golden light in its place. You may "see" or feel the red color of fear in their stomach area, for example, and replace it with cooling green.

9. Trust your intuitions and allow the subtle healing energy to do its work until it seems like time to stop.

10. If your mind wanders during this process, just drop any distracting thoughts, and bring your focus back to what you are doing.

Using your crystals and stones to create emotional change is done *in the present moment*, so as you employ your stones, you must empty your mind, maintain your healing intention, and allow it to happen moment to moment. If your mind wanders into the past or future, focusing on what the emotion *was, how it should* change, or what *it will be like*, the emotional healing will likely not happen. Likewise, if your mind wanders to thoughts about yourself doing the emotional healing rather than merely being a conduit for emotional healing, it will likely not happen.

You can use your crystals to help yourself be entirely present without a wandering mind. Here is a useful method to help you be present-centered:

CRYSTAL MEDITATION TO BE PRESENT-CENTERED

1. Sit upright and hold a clear quartz crystal in each hand with its tip pointing up toward your arm. Surround your body with a circle of smoky quartz crystals with their tips pointing in toward you. If they are larger smoky quartz, you can use four or eight crystals. If smaller, use more. The smaller the crystals, the more you should use so that there is a strong grounding effect to balance any mental activity.

2. Place a rose quartz, pink or green tourmaline, or green malachite over your heart center in the middle of your chest. This stone should be at least 1 to 2 inches in diameter or height.

3. Breathe with long, deep breaths, and imagine that they flow in and out of this heart stone and your heart center. Relax your body with each breath. If your mind wanders, drop your thinking and bring your attention back to your heart center.

4. After at least three minutes, or when you feel centered, silently repeat this to yourself:

5. "I am here now." Do this for at least ten minutes or any length of time. Maintain this state of mind and being as you do your healing work and as you go about your day.

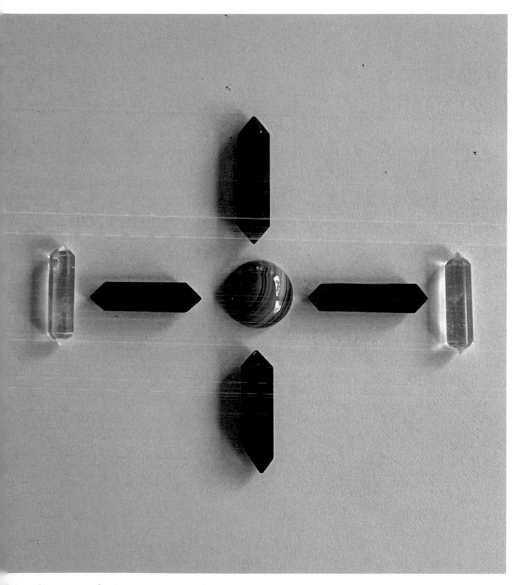

Crystal Layout to be Present-Centered

> NO MATTER WHERE WE ARE,
> WE ARE ALWAYS HERE NOW.
> BE HERE.

It is also important to realize that using your stones to change an emotion isn't something that you *do* to another. Rather, you use your crystals or stones *in partnership* with the other person to *allow* emotional change to happen. Likewise, you can't force an emotion to change within yourself. You can only use your stones to allow it to happen. Think of this as merely using your stones and crystals to set the conditions. Then you "get out of the way" to allow it to happen. To "get out of the way" is to stop thinking about your own ego-self, allowing your mind, body, and feelings to be spacious and empty of expectations.

> EMOTIONAL CHANGES CAN NEVER BE FORCED;
> THEY MUST BE ALLOWED.

QUIET MIND, EXPANDED AWARENESS, AND INTENTION

To be able to effectively discern and change vibratory patterns in the ways discussed above, you must be able to operate from your higher chakras or energy centers so that you can intuitively "see" or sense using your nonlinear, nonrational mind. Using rationality rather than your higher awareness will impede your healing ability because your concrete, rational mind does not bring you the sensitivity needed to feel or sense the vastly more subtle vibratory reality. Being able to employ the know-ingness that comes from an open heart, third eye, or crown chakras is necessary for true success.

The Ultimate Guide to Emotional Healing with Crystals & Stones

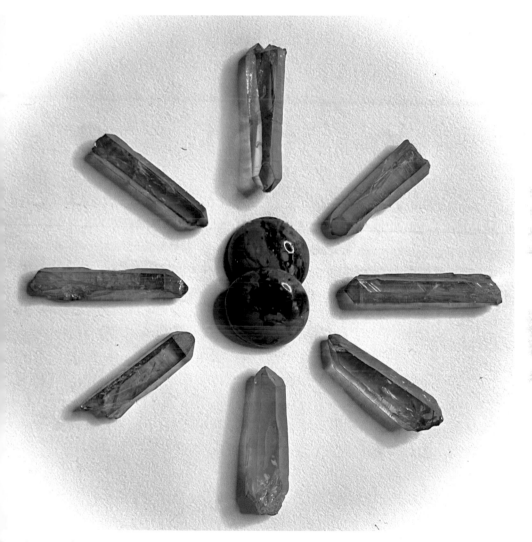

Crystal Layout for a Quiet Mind

QUIET MIND

The rational mind must remain empty of thought to "hear" or sense what the higher centers are saying to you. If your mind is cluttered with thoughts, there is no room for the more subtle ways of knowing to be heard with the "voice" of your inner being. As you do your emotional healing work with your crystals, your mind should be like a clear sky or calm water, open and receptive. The more your mind becomes empty and clear, the more your awareness can expand past the rational mind to access other, more subtle ways of knowing. Whether you "hear" through intuition, psychic sensing, or even more expanded ways of knowing, the information that you receive will be far more accurate. This, of course, vastly improves the effectiveness of your crystal emotional healing work.

An easy way to do this is to regulate your mind with your breath. As you slow your breathing, your mind stops racing and starts emptying of thought. The slower your breath, the calmer your mind. This effect is enhanced if you pay attention to your breathing instead of your thinking. You can use your breath in this way as you are doing your crystal healing so that you can "hear" the directions stemming from your intuitive mind and expanded awareness.

CRYSTAL BREATHING TECHNIQUE FOR A QUIET MIND

1. Sitting upright with your feet flat upon the ground and your hands on your lap facing upward, focus on the tip of your nose.

2. Surround yourself with a circle of turquoise, turquoise amazonite, or other sky-blue crystals that are at least 1 to 2 inches in diameter or length. You may use crystals or tumbled stones. If they are terminated, point the tips in toward you. Hold a sky-blue crystal or tumbled stone in each of your upward-facing palms.

3. Begin to breathe with slow, deep breaths. As you breathe in, feel your breath flow past the tip of your nose and deep into your

lungs. Fill your lungs completely without straining or gasping. Once your lungs are filled, gently let your breath release. Feel its release from your lungs to flow across the tip of your nose.

4. As you do this, release any tension in your body. Let go of any thoughts as they enter your mind, letting your mind be clear, empty, and as expansive as an endless sky.

5. Do this for at least ten minutes or until your mind is completely calm. Continue sitting within this clear consciousness.

This is also a useful practice to do with someone as you work with their emotional healing. If the other person begins to get lost in thoughts of their sadness, anger, anxiety, or other troubling emotion, ask them to take a break and do this breathing practice, letting go of their thoughts in the process. Many times, these negative thoughts are protective in nature, shielding the person from deeper emotional pain. If so, it may be hard for them to let these angry, anxious, or other thoughts go. If so, ask them if it is okay to let these thoughts go temporarily just while they do this practice, telling them that they can always "pick them up" when they are through if they like. (Most of the time, they will have shifted emotionally so much that they don't have the need to "pick up" these thoughts again during the session.)

Opening the Higher Energy Centers

Besides quieting your mind, it is equally important to open your higher energy centers (chakras) to help your awareness expand beyond the rational. When you are centered in your higher energy centers or chakras, you will become increasingly aware of more subtle levels of reality that will bring their information to you. Though the information from your higher energy centers is well beyond rationality, you will find that it makes total sense. You will feel within you a sense of already knowing

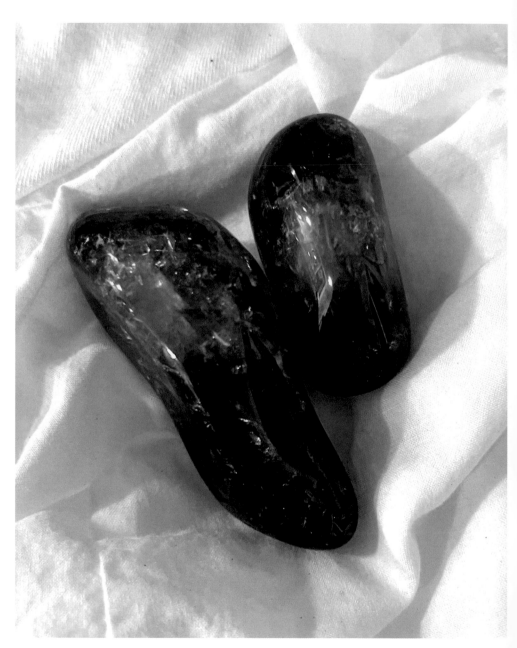

Amethyst Hand Crystals

what you are discerning. It has a sense of familiarity and feels in alignment with your sense of inner truth.

Each higher energy center has its own form of wisdom to give you. The heart is wise in ways that the rational, thinking mind is not. If your third eye is open, you become very intuitive, "hearing" with your inner ear, or "seeing" with your inner eye. It is as if you know without knowing how you know. Like the information received with an open heart, this information is often more accurate than rationality. Your crown chakra, the energy center roughly on the top, center of your head, brings you information from the angelic realms, upward through the heavens into the highest planes of consciousness. There is no good way to describe the source of this timeless wisdom and information that will flow throughout your body, mind, and being. *It is always accurate* if you are open enough with a clear mind devoid of expectations and pre-conceptions. You will always know what to do and how to do it when you refer to this wisdom. If the subtle energy center in your throat (throat chakra) is stimulated and open, you will be able to give accurate and sensitive expression to the wisdom that you receive through these other energy centers. You will always know what to say and when to say it.

Not only is it good to have your upper energy centers open and receptive when you do your crystal emotional healing work, it is also effective to use your crystals to open the higher energy centers of the other person as you work with them. The more their upper energy centers are open, the more they can be receptive to, or "hear," what you are saying to them. They will likely be able to hold their emotional upset in a larger context and learn that their current emotional upset isn't the only reality that is necessarily true for them. They will be able to release what is guarded and repressed considering the larger perspective that they now sense. This expanded awareness can be compared to the difference between being held in a tight box in which their emotions are hugely predominant, to a large room in which their emotions are a very small part, to being out in space, in which their emotions hold only a microscopic sense of importance. The less predominant the emotions are, the less threatening they become and the need to guard against them becomes increasingly less important. In this relaxed, open context, it is much easier to work with and release painful and unhelpful emotional patterns. It is also easier to understand the emotional dynamics that are held in place and to release or change those that are painful and unhelpful.

Yoga and meditation as well as crystal work are all good ways to open your higher energy centers. It works well to be able to use your crystals to raise your and the other's consciousness upward into the upper chakras as you do your emotional healing.

> WHEN DOING AN EMOTIONAL HEALING SESSION,
> SHIFT YOUR ATTENTION TO YOUR HIGHER ENERGY CENTERS
> WHILE KEEPING YOUR HEART OPEN AND RECEPTIVE.

CRYSTAL TECHNIQUE TO OPEN YOUR HIGHER ENERGY CENTERS

1. Lie down on your back or have your client lie on his or her back. Have the legs uncrossed and the arms down by the side of the body with the palms facing upward. Face the head straight forward.
2. Place a green malachite, green tourmaline, green jade, or other green crystal or stone on the heart chakra.
3. Place a smoky quartz or other light brown crystal or stone beneath each foot for the grounding that will facilitate the opening of the upper chakras.
4. Place an amethyst crystal above the crown of the head with its tip pointing upward toward the heavens.

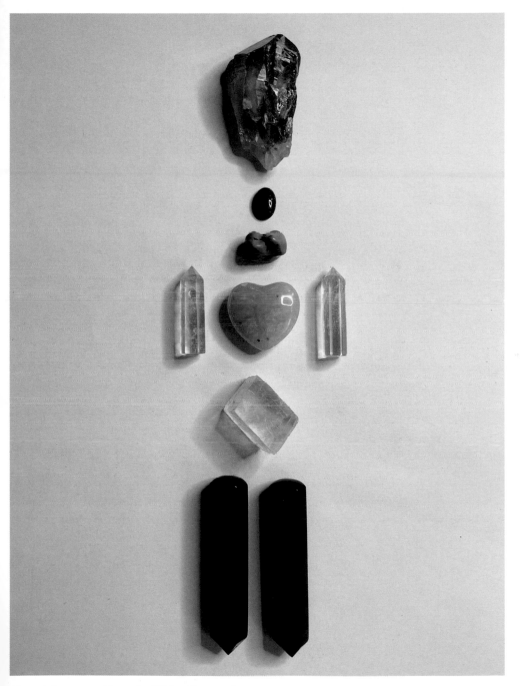

Crystal Layout to Open the Higher Energy Centers

5. After that, place a smaller, light-yellow crystal on the navel center about 2 inches beneath the belly button to help balance and bring the energy necessary to support the opening of the upper energy centers.

6. Place a turquoise stone or crystal in the center of the throat. Make sure it is small enough that it will not put too much pressure on the throat or be uncomfortable.

7. Place a sapphire, lapis, or sodalite on the third eye in the middle of the forehead. If it is a terminated crystal, point the tip upward toward the crown of the head.

8. Hold an amethyst crystal, very bright clear crystal, or Herkimer diamond on the upward palm of each hand. If the stone is single terminated, point its tip upward, facing the arms.

9. Take slow, deep breaths, imagining them flowing in and out of each energy center in this pattern: Breathe in through you heart center and out through your throat center. Then, breathe in through your throat center and out through your third eye. Next, breathe in through your third eye and out through the crown of your head. Continue taking seven more breaths in and out of the energy center in your crown. As you breathe in through these energy centers, imagine that you feel a buzzing sensation or slight breeze stimulating it. Starting with the heart center, repeat this pattern. Do this for at least twenty minutes if you are able.

10. If you find your mind wandering, drop any thoughts that you have and bring your attention back to your breath.

11. If you feel your head tightening, dizziness, or any other constriction, lower your breath to feel as it flows in and out of the bottoms of your feet and relax your body. When this passes, resume the earlier breathing pattern.

Not only can you use this crystal method to help the other person access their higher energy centers during their emotional healing session, but you can use it for yourself, as well. Outside the healing session, you can lie down and place the crystals on your own body and then close your eyes, taking in their energy so that your higher centers open. During an emotional healing session, if you find that you are losing your higher focus, you can quickly and silently take a moment to visualize the crystals on each energy center as you breathe in and out with this breath pattern. You can do this as you continue to listen. Before the session begins, you can place a crystal on your crown center, or your throat, third eye, or heart center, and then do your work. A head band or crystal earrings can be used to stimulate your third eye energy center. A hat or scarf can hold a crystal on your crown. A crystal on a 15- or 16-inch chain can hold a crystal near your throat energy center while a 24-inch chain can hold one on your heart center.

Healing Intention

Not only is it important to be able to have an empty mind devoid of distracting chatter with your attention centered in your higher energy centers, but it is also important to completely concentrate on what you intend to happen during your emotional healing work during your session. This does not mean that you focus on what you imagine the healing outcome should

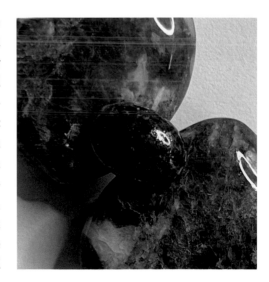

be, or how it should occur, only that emotional healing should occur. As you work with your crystals and stones during the emotional healing session, while maintaining a clear mind without wavering, hold the intention that the emotional healing will happen. In other words, drop your expectancies and let the emotional healing happen as it may. Trust that the emotional healing will happen in the way that is best for the other person, not in the way that is best for your ego. It is helpful to start the emotional healing session with the thought, "Not my way, but Spirit's way." It is entirely possible that the emotional healing will not be like you thought it should be or in the way that you expected. As you do your work, while centering yourself in your higher awareness, let the process unfold at the pace and in the ways that naturally occur, removing your own individual ego from the process.

If you hold your emotional healing intention as you do your work, the healing energy has a clear, unobstructed road to enter and flow through. If you let your attention and intention waver, the healing Spirit finds a road full of obstructions, or no road at all, and the healing might be only partial or not happen at all.

If you are having trouble keeping your mind empty of distractions, expectations, or other thoughts, you can silently chant a simple phrase or mantra as you do your work, while still holding the intention that emotional healing happen. Choose a name for the Higher Spirit or healing energy that has meaning for you. This way not only will your mind remain focused, but your energy will tend to remain centered in your upper energy centers. To further amplify this, feel as if this word or phrase flows outward from your heart center for most of your work. To have it be even more effective, imagine that this word for the healing spirit flows in and out of your third eye in the middle of your forehead or in and out from the top of your head.

The Mind/Body Connection and Placebo Effect

Mind and emotion are intimately related. No feeling remains unaffected by thought, nor does any thought lack an emotional component, even if ever so slight. If you are feeing scared, for example, you will usually have thoughts of what scares you now or what frightened you in the past. You may be consciously or unconsciously reacting to a decision you made in the past that brings you fear in the present. Perhaps you are remembering times when a significant other hit you, for example, and your accompanying unconscious decision that anytime you are with a similar looking person, you will get hit. You may feel fearful, then, every time you are around dark-haired people or persons larger than you. Likewise, you may have thoughts that you are ugly, dumb, or deficient in some way. As a result of these thoughts about yourself, you constantly feel unworthy, sad, or depressed. These conscious and unconscious thoughts don't have to make sense, especially if they are in reaction to long ago occurrences.

When you work with your crystals to help with emotional healing, you shouldn't ignore this mind/body connection. In fact, some very powerful emotional healing work can be done working with this mind/body connection directly. One way is to transform the bodily reactions that support painful emotions. Another way is to change the thoughts that support the emotional trauma.

There are several ways to work with thoughts or the thought patterns that support negative emotions. You can use your crystals to help you intuit the unconscious thoughts that are underlying the emotional upset and work directly to change these thoughts as you verbalize them. You can use your crystals to help someone feel free and safe enough to voice negative thoughts that are conscious and then work to change them. You can use them to bring any hidden thoughts to light by creating a sense of safety and building a different, healthier, perspective.

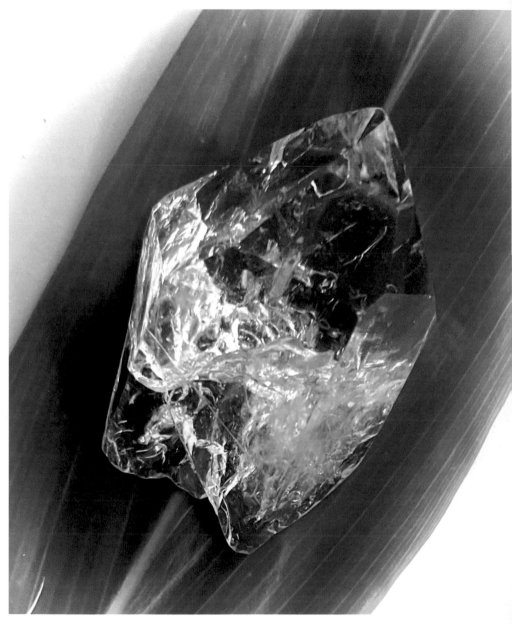

Clear Quartz

Traumatic thought patterns are quite often accompanied by bodily sensations. Or the body will assume various defensive postures or behaviors that are unconsciously designed to protect against troubling emotions. Sitting with a bent posture with the arms wrapped around the stomach or abdomen may reflect fear and be an unconscious protection against its effect. A tight jaw may reflect anger and the need to avoid its expression. Likewise, pressing down on top of the head may be an unconscious expression of a need to avoid an explosion of words or behavior that may result in getting hurt or rejected. During an emotional healing session, it is useful to notice these bodily postures and explore what is revealed when they are released. The same holds true with sensa tions in the body. There may be tightness, pain, 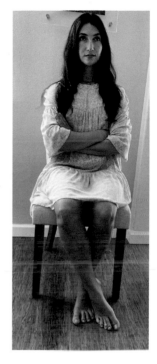 nausea, or uneasiness in certain areas of the body that, when released, reveal difficult emotions. Unconscious feelings of rejection, for example, may manifest as throat pain as tears are blocked. Similarly, feelings of being unloved may manifest in the body as tightness in the chest or pain around the heart area.

In short, working with this mind/body connection can be very powerful in your crystal emotional healing work. Use your expanded awareness to notice these areas of the body. With awareness, you will be able to intuit or even feel in your own body these subtle, physical manifestations of emotional pain. During your emotional healing sessions, then, also pay attention to the positions that the other person assumes with their body as they interact with you and intuit or sense what they mean. Then use techniques to explore and release these positions and sensations to reveal and treat the underlying repressed feelings and thoughts.

Crystals and the Placebo Effect

Very often, crystal work is dismissed as "merely the placebo effect," that the crystals are not doing anything at all, that it is "all in the mind." It could be said that all in existence is merely a reflection of mind because of the mind/body connection, so in that sense, the change we make with our crystals truly is mentally related. However, this understanding shouldn't be used to dismiss crystal healing work. Because of the placebo effect and the mind/body interaction, one way to look at crystal work, instead, is that we use our crystals to skillfully manipulate the placebo effect. We can use our crystals to help change the mind to change the mental/emotional/physical condition. We can use our crystals to help us expand our awareness and release the limitations that we impose upon ourselves with our beliefs and expectations so that we are happier. Ultimately, it is important to realize that the crystal is just a tool, an effective tool, but still a tool. The crystal does not do the healing. Spirit heals.

SECTION THREE
ABOUT EMOTIONS

It is not enough to just place a crystal on someone who is suffering emotionally and expect the troubling emotions to magically pass. Though there may be some initial placebo effect accompanied by wishful thinking, any effects are generally going to be quite minimal without any lasting effect.

This is not to say that it doesn't work at all to just place crystals on the body without accompanying them with any other techniques. They can be used as reminders, especially when placed on the body after an emotional healing session. A rose quartz worn on the heart chakra can remind you to shift your attention to the love in your heart every time that you feel ready to explode with anger. It can remind you that not only are you loved, but that in essence, you are love itself. A crystal placed on your forehead can remind you to relax your mind whenever it seems about to be overtaken with anxious thoughts. Even carrying a quartz crystal can remind you that beneath all confusing and troubling emotions is crystal clarity and ease. It is especially powerful to use the crystals in this way after an emotional healing session to help carry on and deepen the work that you did while there. However, emotional healing with your crystals works best when you also use them with accompanying techniques that address all the layers of emotion, from the simple to the complex.

Surface Emotions

Emotional upset can range from the simple and temporary to those that are quite complex. More superficial and temporary emotional troubles

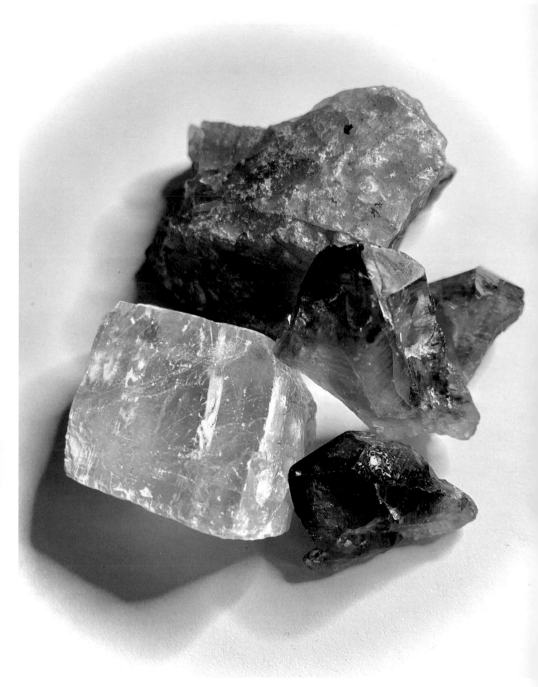

Rose Quartz, Green Calcite, and Amethyst Healing Crystals

are rather easy to help heal, as they are generally based on things that have currently occurred. If you feel ignored or slighted, for example, you may feel sad. However, it may only take a single session to understand the slight and your reaction to it and to remove or change the sadness.

These more superficial emotions are often transitory, appearing and disappearing without any deep effect on your life or sense of being-ness. Crystal work for these more superficial emotional upsets involves helping the person discover that their emotions appear and disappear in their mind and that they are never permanent, even if it appears to be the same feeling. Underneath these endlessly changing emotional states exists a clear, calm state of being upon which these feelings appear and disappear. If you shift your focus from the constantly changing feelings to the space between them, you will eventually discover this calm and clear state.

Deep Emotional Wounding

In contrast, deeper, persistent layers of emotional wounding take a lot more time and care to help heal, requiring many repeated sessions. This is because the initial core wound is subconsciously covered by successive layers of emotion that protect the re-experiencing of the feelings associated with the original, extremely painful, deep emotional injury. Like the peeling of an onion, these deep layers of emotion must be skillfully addressed one by one so that lasting change can occur. It is important to use great care and wisdom as you employ your crystals to discover and heal each emotional layer. This must be done without allowing a new protective layer to form itself. In other words, you use your crystals in techniques that help you move even deeper into the psyche as you reveal each succeeding layer to finally reveal the core emotion. Then you carefully, consciously, lovingly, and skillfully help heal the core emotional wound upon which the others protectively shield.

This process may be frustrating as you do your emotional healing work because often your progress may not be straightforward, but instead may slide backward time after time because of the persistent wounding not releasing easily. The person you are working with may seem to not understand or become unwilling to do the necessary work because of the fright associated with the wounding. It is important to remember that this is part of the process and not make them wrong or blame them for "not trying." Have compassion and remember that they are doing the best they can. It is okay, and in fact, part of the usual process is to repeat a particular healing over and over until, with insight and acceptance, a permanent emotional healing occurs.

Because of the depth and persistence of this emotional wound, it very likely has become ingrained as a deep belief and experience of their self, so to shift the emotion is to shift the very definition and experience of their essential selfhood. As the core emotions shift and the original wounding starts to be held in a new context, it is not unusual to face questions like "Who am I without this wounding?" There is a new space of clarity, of pure beingness, that lacks easy definition and may, thus, be quite uncomfortable for the person who has been healed. If this is the case, you must help the healed person relax and be at ease in this new spaciousness and new sense of pure self. By changing the debilitating emotion or emotional patterns, you are helping bring about a new and life-changing sense of self for the healed person.

Typical Core Wounds

The emotions that are more superficial and those that result from early core wounds are the same ones you are used to seeing: fear, anger, hate, aversion, contempt, disgust, and so on. The difference is both in their intensity and their persistence. The feelings associated with core wound-ing feel overwhelming, so big that you can't do anything about them and

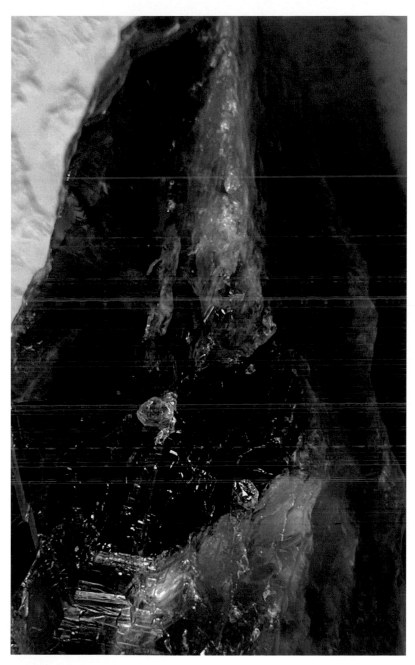

Amethyst

you are totally in their control. To manage them, or avoid feeling them at all, you can get sick, project them outward to others so that they don't seem to be yours, get depressed, deeply anxious, or confused. You may develop obsessive behaviors to attempt their control. You may even feel that they are so big that you will die from them or that you want to die. In short, they can feel so huge that you become afraid of experiencing them, so afraid, in fact, that you will do almost anything not to feel them.

Early Childhood Events, Conclusions, and Emotional Wounding

These deep emotional wounds are so pervasive and debilitating because they are in response to events that happened to you when you were very young and vulnerable, often pre-verbal. Basically, they are based on the perception of the withdrawal of love from a significant other, parent, or caregiver upon whom you are totally dependent for love and for your own survival. The natural reaction to this perceived abandonment or withdrawal of love is to get angry at the one doing this to you. However, if you get angry at the parent, significant other, or caretaker, you risk losing their love even more and this is extremely frightening on the most basic level, seeming to risk your very survival. To understand and handle this seemingly catastrophic loss of love and abandonment that threatens to leave you alone, scared, and vulnerable in the world, you react to it or understand it by unconsciously or consciously blaming yourself instead of the parent or caretaker, deciding that something is fundamentally wrong with you. These pre-verbal decisions are made so unconsciously and buried so deeply within your psyche that you don't even remember making them.

The caretaker may not have even done what you think was done to you. Or it may have been in reaction to a careless moment or communication on the parent's or caretaker's part that seemed so unimportant or fleeting that they, themselves, don't even remember it. To you, however,

The Ultimate Guide to Emotional Healing with Crystals & Stones

it was momentous, negatively changing your self-perception in ways that cause extreme emotional pain. In your pre-reasoning mind, however, it is better that you feel pain rather than lose the caretaker upon whom you so depend for your life and essential nurturance. If they abandon you, the pre-verbal mind reasons, you will die. This is frightening.

This is not to say that these early actions by the parent, significant other, or caretaker never took place or that the abuse that you experienced at this early life stage never really took place. Unfortunately, it is often true that it did. Whether the actions took place or not, it is your perception and reaction that is important because you still carry its effect within you as reoccurring and pervasive deep emotional wounding.

The following are some of the most typical forms of early childhood events and the conclusions reached by the child: When the parent or caretaker withdraws his or her love, for example, the child typically makes the decision that they are basically unlovable. If the loved one or significant other rejects the child, her or she then decides that people will always leave them. If the child suffered rape, violence, or any form of personal violation, for example, they may make the decision that they can never trust anyone. If the child suffers betrayal from a loved one, for example, the resulting decision may be that they are deficient in some way or that something is fundamentally wrong with him or her. If the child feels engulfed, or that his or her individuality is smothered by the parent or caretaker, the child may feel that the resulting anger will risk losing the parent. Similarly, if the child is manipulated by a loved one, or if they are being used by the parent or caretaker to fulfill their own needs instead of the child's, the resulting decision may be that they are fundamentally unworthy.

These are only some of the typical types of decisions that can be made. However, no matter what the decision, it involves turning on or invalidating themselves and the emotional result is anger, despair, shame, grief, guilt, distrust, apathy, or contempt. Sometimes the person feels more than one of these feelings.

There is more to this dynamic, however. Because these feelings about themselves are so painful to bear, the person then, more often than not, further reacts in a way to distance themselves from having to experience these, as well. Fundamental anger may be covered by blame. Depression may be a reaction to apathy or grief. Disgust for other people may cover a deep sense of shame.

Another typical reaction is to project these reactive feelings outward so that instead of feeling them themself, the person experiences others as having them. Instead of feeling their own anger, for example, they experience everyone else as being angry and then react accordingly. Instead of their own fundamental feeling of guilt, for example, they experience other people as always doing things wrong, or as never living up to their own expectations of perfection. If their fundamental feeling is one of distrust, for example, they may, in turn, lie or cheat because "everyone is doing it" or to "get a jump" on people. Or they may feel constantly anxious.

In reaction to these feelings, then, it is not unusual for the emotional layering to continue. To cover up their suicidal feelings, for example, they may decide to "keep a happy face" and be artificially happy all the time. Then, in reaction to this fake happiness, they may feel pressure and exhaustion, which expresses itself as depression. Thus, the emotional layering continues. (These typical core wounds, their emotional reactions, and ways to heal them are explained in detail later in this book.)

When working to heal deep emotional wounding, then, you must first start with the most outward layer of emotion to reach what is deeper. As was expressed earlier, this must be done carefully, because each layer covers up and defends against deeper feelings. In the above case, for example, if you just treat the depression or try to make it go away, you may miss the emotional exhaustion underneath. The likely result is that the person will come up with another feeling to handle it, perhaps with overeating or another eating disorder, for example.

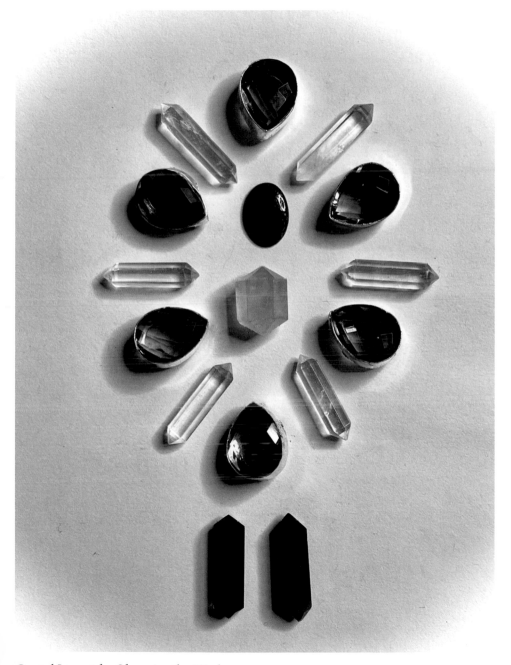

Crystal Layout for Observing the Mind

Meditations and Practices to Help

To help yourself or another person be free of the transitory negative emotions, you can use your crystals along with these three simple practices. You can use these techniques also for the deeper, core emotional wounding to help peel away each emotional layer, employing other accompanying techniques as well. (These other techniques will be explained later.)

OBSERVING THE MIND

1. Sit upright in a straight-backed chair or in lotus or half lotus yoga position with your head facing forward.
2. Surround your body with alternating royal blue and clear quartz crystals or tumbled stones. If terminated, point their tips in toward the body.
3. Hold a lapis, sodalite, blue quartz, or other royal blue crystal or stone in each hand. If they are terminated, point the tips upward toward the arms so that they are both receptive.
4. Place or wear a lapis, sodalite, or royal blue sapphire on your third eye. For more empowerment, also wear these stones or crystals as earrings.
5. Place or wear a rose quartz, pink tourmaline, rhodochrosite, or solid pink rhodonite on your heart center.
6. Place smoky quartz or a light brown crystal or tumbled stone beneath each foot so that you are grounded and empowered.
7. Focus on your heart center, breathe with gentle, deep breaths, and imagine that each breath passes in and out of your heart center. As you do this, allow your body to relax. Do this for three minutes or until you feel centered and relaxed.
8. Shift your attention to your third eye in the middle of your forehead. Relax your forehead.

The Ultimate Guide to Emotional Healing with Crystals & Stones

9. With your energy centered in your forehead, notice your thoughts. (Your first thought that you notice might be "What thought?" Notice that thought first.) Notice each thought as it comes to you. Notice that each thought appears and then disappears. This is true even if it is a recurring thought. Watch this progression of thoughts for at least ten minutes at first, then twenty minutes or longer as you are able. If your mind wanders, notice these thoughts. As you get started, you might notice thoughts like, "This is boring." Or "I can't do this." "I'm tired of doing this." If so, notice these thoughts also.

10. After you are completely focused on your thoughts as they come and go, notice that there is an empty space between each thought. Focus on that empty space. Notice that thoughts seem to appear from this space and disappear into this space. Do this for another ten to twenty minutes, or as long as you are able.

11. When you are finished, remove each crystal in the reverse order in which you set it out and energetically clear each one. Arise from your sitting position.

Though this meditation is simple, it can be quite powerful and healing. This meditation will help you realize that there is no such thing as a "stuck" thought. All thoughts, negative or positive, appear and disappear in the underlying clear space of your mind. As you go about your day, any time you feel stuck in negativity or engulfed in painful emotions, notice the thoughts that accompany these feelings, and then notice that these feelings come and go. Just as thoughts have spaces between them, the painful emotions do also. They are not all-encompassing. Rather than focusing on and allowing yourself to be vulnerable to the re-occurring, painful emotions, pay attention to the spaciousness or clear, empty space within which they are held. Focus on this space and you will find that your negative emotions start losing their power until they seem to pass entirely.

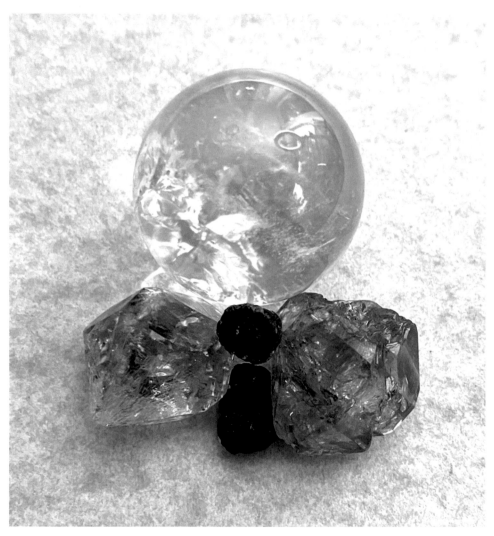

Crystal Layout to Release Negative Emotions

CRYSTAL VISUALIZATION TO RELEASE NEGATIVE EMOTIONS

1. Sit upright in front of a large, very clear, single terminated quartz crystal or crystal ball at eye level. Place it about 12 inches from your body. The diameter of the crystal ball should be at least 2 inches. The clear quartz should be at least 3 inches high and 2 inches wide with one of its six faces pointing directly at you.

2. Place a clear quartz crystal or Herkimer diamond in each hand to empower this visualization. They should be the same type of crystal in each hand. If you are using single terminated crystals, point the tip of the left-hand crystal toward your arm in receptive position. Point the tip of the one in your right hand outward in manifesting position.

3. Place a royal-blue colored crystal on your third eye or wear royal-blue crystal earrings. This will activate your third eye to empower and make it easier to visualize. It will also help you release negative emotions.

4. After centering and grounding yourself, gaze into the crystal or crystal ball in front of you. Find a place that interests you or draws your attention. Bring all your focus to that area.

5. Investigate that area further and further, seeing more and more detail. If your mind wanders, bring it back to the crystal and resume your exploration. Look deeper into the crystal until you are unaware of anything else. Eventually you will feel as if you are inside the crystal. Then let your eyes close.

6. Imagine yourself as sitting inside the crystal in a chair with a big bag next to you. Then, feel the emotion that you want to change. As you feel this emotion, imagine that you place it in the bag next to you. Continue placing all the negative emotions in the bag until you feel no more of them.

7. Imagine that you tie the top of the bag so that the emotions stay inside. After that, imagine that the bag becomes like a balloon and begins to lift off from the ground beside you. Imagine that it lifts further and further until it becomes a little dot that eventually you can't see at all. As it floats away, you feel mentally calm, your mind light and free.

8. Sitting calmly in your chair, take a deep breath and gently blow it out. Do this three times. Each time your mind feels more and more free, and you feel happy. Rest with this feeling for as long a time as you like.

9. When you are ready, notice the chair you are sitting on. Now, notice the crystal around you until you eventually see its edge. Imagine that you see a door open at the edge of the crystal. Then imagine getting up from the chair and leaving through the door.

10. As you leave through the door, imagine that you see the crystal in front of you, and as you watch, it gets smaller and smaller until it sits in front of you. Become aware of the chair upon which you sit and feel the ground beneath your feet. When you are ready, open your eyes and get up. See if you can continue through your day with your clear and restful mind.

USING YOUR CRYSTAL TO REMOVE TROUBLING EMOTIONS

This is a crystal practice that you can easily do in an emotional healing session or just during your day if you notice troubling feelings appear. You can easily do this for yourself as well as with other people. This technique works well with the more superficial emotions. It also works well with deep-seated core emotional wounds if you use it to remove each layer of wounding, one by one.

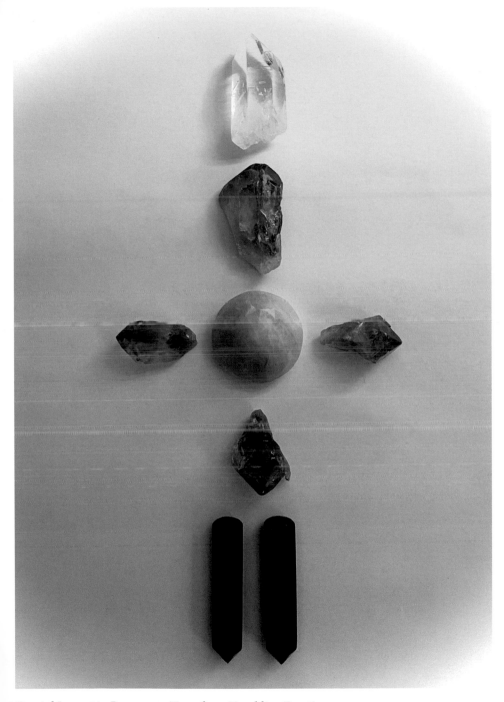

Crystal Layout to Remove or Transform Troubling Emotions

USING YOUR CRYSTALS TO REMOVE OR TRANSFORM EMOTIONS

1. Hold a clear, single terminated quartz crystal in your right hand. It should be at least 2 inches in height and 1 inch in width and be clear rather than cloudy or dull so that it has the power for this technique.

2. Hold an amethyst in your left hand to help channel in the higher awareness needed for transformative wisdom. This crystal should be approximately 2 inches in height and 1 inch in width. It can be single or double terminated. If single terminated, point its tip up toward your arm to channel its energy inward.

3. If you are doing this for yourself, wear a pink crystal on your heart chakra in the middle of your chest. If you are doing this for someone else, have them lie down flat on their back, hands upward in receptive position, and surround their body with amethyst crystals. Place a grounding smoky quartz or brown-colored crystal beneath their feet and a clear crystal over their head with the tip pointing outward. Place a rose quartz, pink tourmaline, or other pink crystal on their heart center to help open their heart center, the seat of the emotions.

4. Breathe with long, deep breaths in and out of the heart center. If you are assisting another, also breathe in and out of your heart center until you feel centered and grounded.

5. After becoming grounded and centered, have the other person or yourself focus on the troubling emotion that they would like to have transformed. Try to experience it in its entirety. Where does it seem to be centered in your body? Usually, you will find it centered in the head, throat, stomach, or mid-chest. What color do you imagine this emotion to be? What temperature? If this negative emotion had a voice, what would it say? Ask yourself or the other these and any other pertinent questions about the emotion so that you can experience it completely.

6. As the emotion is being described, open yourself to receive this information. Imagine it entering the amethyst crystal in your left hand to bring you even more clarity about it. If you are working with another, let yourself feel this emotion in your own body and psyche so that you become completely familiar with it.

7. Once the emotion has been experienced as completely as possible, use the clear crystal in your right hand to "scoop out" or cut out the negative emotion each place that it is felt. As you do this, point the tip of your crystal to the earth and imagine that this negative emotion, in the form of gray light, flows into the earth where it is transmuted to positivity. Imagine that the gray light transforms to light green light as it is transmuted. As you draw this negative emotion from the other, feel as if it also travels out of yourself into the earth. Once all the gray, negative emotional energy is removed from an area, then send in its opposite energy in the form of rose, then amethyst light. Do this for yourself or the other.

8. As you are removing the negative, troubling emotion, ask the other to feel the opposite, more positive emotion as you are removing the negative. If they are having trouble doing that, ask them to *imagine* feeling a more positive emotion in the same area from which you are drawing the negativity out. As they do this, hold the amethyst crystal over that area or point it toward the area and imagine amethyst light filling it with positivity and healing.

9. Another option is to ask them what color that new, positive emotion might be, and then send in that color light with the same color crystal. If, for example, they imagine that their sadness is now happiness and imagine the associated color to be yellow as the sun, use a yellow jade, yellow citrine, or other yellow crystal to send in its light. If the person is lying on their back in receptive

position, you can place this crystal on this area and leave it there during the session.

10. Ask if there is any other area in the body in which they feel this negative, emotional upset. If they can't feel any other area, ask them *to imagine* where else they may feel this gray, negative energy. Repeat the same process in this new area, drawing out the gray, negative emotional energy and replacing it with amethyst or any associated color and colored crystal.

11. Keep doing this until there seem to be no more places that this painful, negative emotional energy is felt or imagined.

12. If you are doing this for yourself, have a collection of colored crystals near you that you can use for this process, one by one, sending their energy into your body.

13. Once you are through, have the other person rest comfortably with the various colored crystals on their body while breathing in and out of their heart center with long, deep, gentle breaths. As they do this, ask them to visualize themselves being surrounded in an amethyst aura of light, or an aura of light that matches the color stones on their body. As they continue breathing with long, deep breaths, ask them to relax into this aura of emotionally healing light, letting it fill them body, heart, mind, and soul. If you are doing this for yourself, let yourself similarly relax within an aura of healing amethyst or colored crystal light. This relaxation period should be for at least 11 minutes, if not longer. Gently and softly remind the other of this crystal light around their body to bring back a wondering mind or to keep them from falling asleep.

14. When through, gently remove the various crystals on the body and place aside the clear and amethyst crystals in your hand. Use the smoke of sage, cedar, or other clearing herbs to sweep the body from head to toe, re-balancing and clearing them of any

lingering negativity. Also sweep yourself with this smoke from head to toe, imagining that any "stuck" energy leaves through the bottom of your feet into the earth where it is transmuted to positivity. Do this until you feel completely clear.

15. Clear your crystals and wrap them until you use them again for another emotional healing session.

As you do this process, you will likely find that emotions that seem so "stuck" are not as persistent or "solid" as you think. Even the most pervasive emotion has spaces within it. They appear and disappear, even though it may be so fleeting as to be beyond conscious awareness. The more you quiet your mind, deepen your perception, and expand your consciousness so that you are aware of more and more emotional subtlety, the more that you will experience that the negative emotion doesn't quite have you in the grip you think it does. Your work is to expand these spaces of clarity. Your quiet mind, and your ability to expand the space of emotional clarity, will get stronger the longer you do this emotional healing process.

EMOTIONS ARE NOT AS SOLID AND UNMOVEABLE AS WE THINK THEY ARE. FOCUS ON THE SPACES WITHIN EACH EMOTIONAL THOUGHT PATTERN.

An important thing to keep in mind when doing this process of emotional removal is that sometimes it can be quite fearful to have a negative emotion removed. There are many reasons for this: Quite a bit of someone's identity could be wrapped up in their negative emotion. If they consciously or subconsciously identify themselves as a depressed person, for example, as painful as it is, it is at least something that they can rely on about themselves. As unhappy as it may make them feel, it offers a familiar feeling and self-definition. If you take away the depression, they may be left with an unknown part of their self, a "hole" in their very center, that they may not know how to fill. If not their depressed self, what or who are they now? This can be very fundamentally frightening.

Another thing to realize about troubling emotions is that, as painful as they are, they can be a way to make you feel unique and special. Again, this is a question of fundamental self-identity. "I am more depressed than anyone else." "No one has ever experienced my depression like I do." "My depression is so bad that there is nothing that you or anyone else can do about it." Though these defensive conclusions cause pain, on a very deep level it gives you a skewed sense of self-worth. If so, it will be very hard to break through this defensive shell since, again, it is a challenge to an entire identity of self.

If the person's identity is partially or completely supported by their painful emotion or emotional pattern, as you work to remove the troubling emotion, there may be tremendous resistance. The other person may not be able to "find" the emotion in their body or imagine a color. They may get angry or in some way strike out at you as you attempt to remove the troubling, yet familiar, feeling. They may deny that they really have it, or let you know that it's "not that bad." They may let you know that there is nothing you can do to help them or that they are beyond help. In the case of depression, for example, their response may be vague when asked where it seems to be centered in their body or they may tell you that they are "only a little sad now and then," despite the fact they came for an emotional healing of that very same feeling. They may tell you that you don't know what you are doing, or that you can't possibly understand how depressed they are since you are not depressed. They may become very angry and even yell and scream at you.

It is important to experience these as defensive behaviors rather than take them personally. It is also important to know that if someone has a severe reaction, it is a manifestation of core wounding and that the particular emotion you are working on is multi-layered. If so, you will need to know how to work around the defenses and work with core wounding. (Never work to remove an emotion if you are not asked to help!) No matter how outlandish their claims are, no matter how they may have attacked you, you are quite aware of their feelings and they are trusting you to carry on.

As you are working to remove these feelings, remember that you are also working with the mind. There are ways to "trick" the mind, to go around defensive thoughts. If the other person, for example, says that they cannot feel where the emotion is in their body, ask that they *imagine* where the feeling is. If they show resistance to letting go of a feeling, let them know that they only have to do it *right now as you are doing the healing*, that they can "pick up" this feeling after the session if they want to.

To keep the other's trust, it is important never to make them wrong in any way. Your job, after all, is to support the process however it unfolds. If the other person lets you know, for example, that they are not feeling sad when you clearly experience that they are, instead of saying, "you're clearly sad" or "you're mistaken," you might say, "If you were feeling sad, where would you feel it?" Or if someone is getting angry with you as you get close to a deep feeling, you may respond with the acknowledgment, "I see that you are angry." And then go further. "Is there anyone else that you are angry with?" or "Tell me how you are feeling. Describe the anger to me. Where do you feel it in your body? or "Are you willing for it to go?" Don't even ask the other person why they are angry. They may not know at that moment.

In short, go where the emotional healing takes you. You may intend to work with depression, for example, yet if anger comes up, then work with that. Ask their permission any time you want to start working with a new feeling other than the one that they initially presented you with. For example, you may ask, "Are you willing to let this anger go, at least for now?" If you find that you end up working with a different emotion than you and the other person initially intended, then ask if they want another session to work with the initial emotion.

It is important to always leave the other person you are working with in as good an emotional space as you can. Even if a session ends up being difficult, let the other know that it is time to end the session and then do the work to get them balanced, grounded, and peaceful. Have them lie down with amethyst around their body and rose quartz on their heart chakra and breathe with long, deep breaths in and out of their heart chakra in the middle of their chest. Ask them to imagine letting all their troubling feelings go and relax their body more with each breath. Clear their aura or energetic body with the smoke of sage, cedar, or any herb that draws you and them. Blow or sweep down from head to toe, having them imagine any negativity leaving through the bottoms of their feet into the earth as you do this. Then have them imagine an aura of clear, golden light surrounding their body.

As with any crystal healing work, be sure to ground, clear, and center yourself as well so that you do not have any negative energy left in you that you may have drawn in.

KEEP YOUR HEALING CENTERED IN THE MOMENT
EVEN IF/WHEN RECALLING PAST EVENTS.
HOW ARE YOU FEELING NOW?

SECTION FOUR
CRYSTAL AND STONE EMOTIONAL HEALING KIT

The following are the most basic crystals and stones that you will need to do an effective job with emotional healing. Each crystal or stone is named and described, along with the emotional healing work they are generally used for. Though the heart crystals and stones are generally the most important to have, you will find that you will need to combine them with other crystals for protection, communication, insight, and trust. As you do your emotional healing work, you will find that no one of these types of crystals stands alone but are combined with each other to accentuate and accelerate the healing process. To open the heart center, for example, you need an accompanying sense of protection to safely be able to express your wants and needs. You will also need to combine it with a grounding crystal to provide this help. The person you are working with may also be unable to find the words to express what they are feeling. To help with this, you may also need to add a crystal that works with communication.

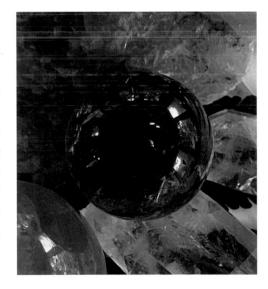

Here is a list of the crystals and stones for your emotional healing kit followed by a few other crystals or stones that you may want to have to fine-tune or address the deeper subtleties of your work. The primary crystals and stones, the ones that you should have in your kit, are first described along with the number of them you should have. They are divided into the following categories: 1.) the two most essential crystals; 2.) the heart crystals; 3.) the protection and grounding crystals; 4.) the communication crystals; and 5.) the insight crystals. Before the list and descriptions of stones and their uses, important information about each of these categories is described along with some accompanying emotional healing techniques. When it is not necessary to have all the different crystals or stones in each category, it will be noted in the text. Following the list of the primary crystals and stones, additional or secondary crystals are enumerated. These are not absolutely necessary for you to have but are useful crystals and stones to finetune your work.

Crystal and Stone Emotional Healing Kit

CATEGORY, NUMBER & SIZES
TWO MOST IMPORTANT
Clear Quartz 2 large, 10 small, 2 Herkimer diamonds
Amethyst 2 large, 10 small

HEART CRYSTALS
Rose Quartz 1 large, 2 medium, 8 small
Pink Tourmaline 1 large, 4 small
Pink Calcite 1 large, 2 medium, 4 small
Pink Coral, M. O. P., Pearl 8 small

PROTECTION CRYSTALS
Black Tourmaline 1 large, 4 small
Black Onyx 4 medium or small
Black Agate 4 medium or small
Smoky Quartz 1 large, 10 small
Yellow Citrine 2 small to medium
Yellow Jade 2 small to medium
Yellow Calcite 2 small to medium

COMMUNICATION CRYSTALS
Turquoise 4 small
Aqua Aura 1 large
Larimar 3 small

INSIGHT CRYSTALS
Lapis Lazuli 1 small to medium
Blue Sodalite 1–2 small to medium
Blue Azurite 1 small
Blue Sapphire 1–4 small

ADDITIONAL/ SECONDARY
Green Malachite 1 medium
Green Calcite 1 medium
Blue Lace Agate 2 small
White Howlite 2 small
Lepidolite 1 large
Garnet 1 medium to large
Amber 1 medium to large

OTHER VIOLET CRYSTALS
Purple Charoite 1 small
Purple Sugilite 1 small
Purple Tanzanite 1 small
Purple Iolite 1 small
Purple Fluorite 4 medium

Clear Quartz Crystals

Clear quartz is one of the most important crystals to have in your emotional healing kit. They are natural energy amplifiers and as such can be placed on any energy center to stimulate and open it when you don't have an appropriately colored crystal to use. Even better, a clear quartz crystal can be used to increase the effects of any colored stone by placing it alongside or on top of the colored crystal or stone as you use it. Though it is best to have the actual colored crystal to use, if you don't, you can program the clear quartz with that color and then use it as you would use the colored stone itself. (See *The Ultimate Guide to Crystal Healing* to learn how to program clear crystals.) Since the power of the programming is only as strong as your powers of concentration, it is generally better to have the actual colored stone. As has been demonstrated earlier in this book, you can use the clear crystal to manipulate subtle energy to do your healing work. Again, this can be quite useful for augmenting the healing work that your colored crystals and stones are doing as they are laid on the body.

The clearer and brighter a quartz crystal is, the more powerful its energy is. Size is not as important as clarity. The quartz crystals have points on one end, called single terminated, or on each end, called double terminated. The flow of the energy is outward through its tip. Be sure to use natural quartz crystals rather than lab-created. They are more

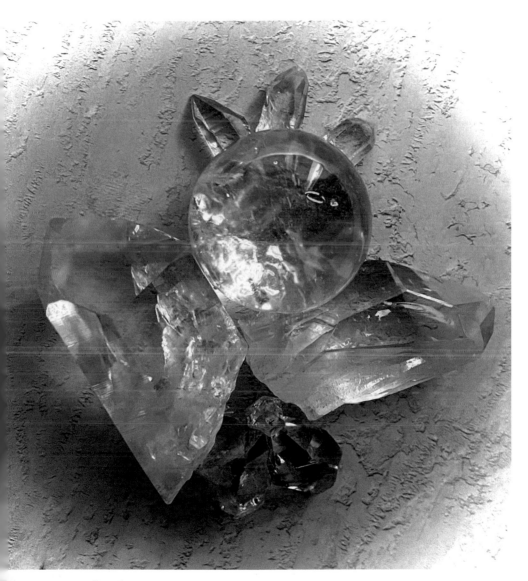

Clear Quartz and Herkimer Diamonds

powerful. Some synthetic crystals are plastic or just glass; they are pretty but can't do this type of energy work. Some people prefer a natural, untouched quartz crystal while others prefer a cut and polished natural quartz crystal. Both will work, although if the polished quartz crystal was not cut along the natural lines through which its energy flows, it will not work very well. To be sure that the energy is flowing properly, hold the crystal in your left hand and meditate with it. If you aren't sure, use raw, natural quartz crystals.

You should have two single terminated clear crystals at least 3 inches high and 1 inch wide with their tips intact. Your emotional healing kit should also have at least ten small, single-terminated clear quartz crystals that are at least 1.5 inches in length with single terminations so that you can use them to surround the body, place on each energy center, or other amplifying uses. It is also good to have at least one very clear Herkimer diamond approximately 0.75 inches in height. Herkimer diamonds, the most powerful of all quartz crystals, are very good for working with the highest energy centers, including the third eye and crown.

Amethyst Crystals

Amethyst is also vitally important to have in your crystal and stone emotional healing kit. Amethysts are the "workhorses" of all healing work. They help enable all types of healing, whether it's physical, mental, or emotional. If you aren't sure what color crystal or stone to use with an emotional healing issue, use amethyst.

Amethyst is an upper energy center crystal. It is used to energize and open the subtle energy center above your head associated with higher "cosmic" consciousness. When this center is open, it will lift your awareness beyond the physical into the metaphysical and spiritual. It will help you gain the information from these realms to help you in your emotional healing work. It will help lift someone out of their emotional turmoil to give them a larger, more peaceful perspective.

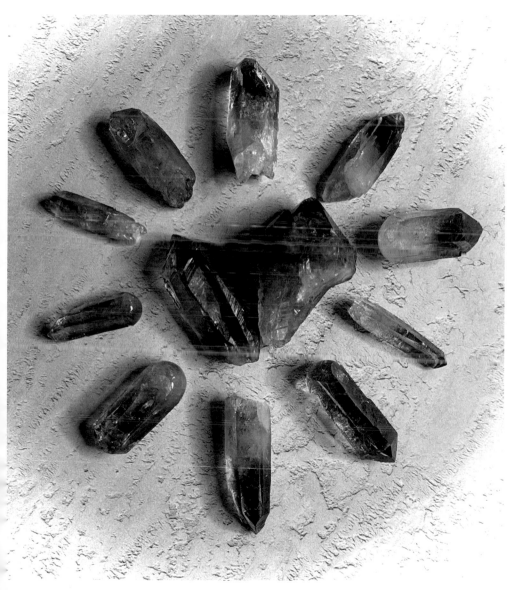

Amethyst for Emotional Healing Kit

Your emotional healing kit should include at least two single-terminated amethysts that are at least 2 inches long and 1 inch wide. You should also have at least ten other smaller single-terminated amethysts approximately and 1.25 inches long and a 0.5 inches wide. Like the clear quartz, this will give you enough amethyst to use on all of the body's energy centers or do any other emotional healing technique. You can use ten tumbled amethysts instead of the single terminated crystals. However, if you use tumbled, though you still have the amethyst energy to work with, you will not be able to direct the energy flow in or out of the body like you can when the amethyst has terminations.

Heart Crystals and Stones

Crystals for the heart center, of course, are used the most in emotional healing work. All emotions, both pleasant and unpleasant, pleasurable or painful, reside in and are reflected in the heart center. Since emotions are centered in the heart, difficult and painful emotions usually result in a partially closed or entirely closed heart center. With a closed heart center, you may experience a lack of compassion for others and yourself. You may lack the empathy to understand and accept others and often become demanding and impatient. With a closed heart center, you may be unable to experience true intimacy since such feelings demand openness toward others as well as yourself. The more your heart is closed, the less you can feel love. If so, your love can become demanding and you may feel angry as you fail to experience the love that you expect. You may feel sad without a sense of being loved or understood, feel despair in its place, or feel that there must be something innately unlovable about you, failing to understand how you are contributing to this. All these feelings and more are a sign of a closed heart center.

Not only will a closed heart center have emotional effects, but it will likely also have mental and physical effects. Your physical heart may become ill or have other problems, or your chest muscles may painfully constrict as you try to stop having the painful feelings. Your back muscles

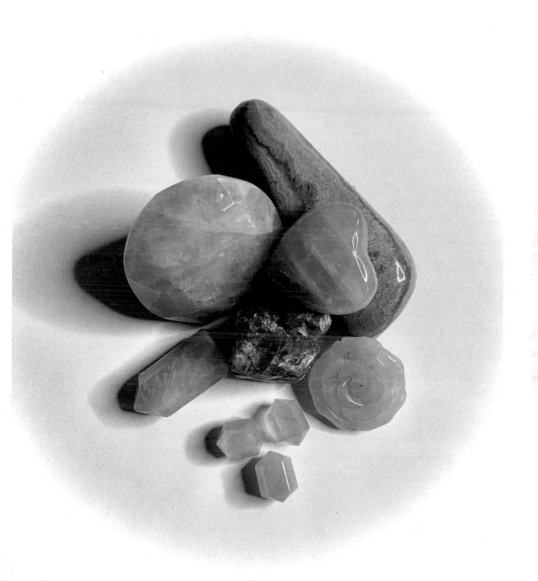

Rose Quartz, Rhodochrosite, and Pink Tourmaline Heart Healing Crystals

may become tight as they couple with your restricted chest muscles. This constriction may start to misalign your spine and have effects on the organs associated with the heart, including your lungs. Your breathing may become constricted and your throat sore.

Since the emotions and mind are related, each affecting the other, you may find yourself hating or strongly disliking specific people who you perceive as not caring about you, or all people in general. Your mental experience of the world is not pleasant, and according to your thinking, the world is a hateful, hostile place where other people only care about themselves. These thoughts, in turn, increase your sense of emotional isolation and close your heart even further.

When you begin to open the heart center, you are likely going to also work with physical and mental healing. Even though you experience the mental and physical effects of a closed heart, know that these ramifications will likely heal to the extent that the heart opens and emotional healing takes place. This does not mean that you or the other person should ignore physical effects. There is a time to go to the doctor or psychiatrist. However, you can always do your emotional healing work in conjunction with the work that these people do. If someone in your care becomes truly suicidal, it is completely necessary for that to be reported to a suicide prevention line or other appropriate people.

You will be able to use your crystals coupled with your intuition and higher awareness to feel or sense if the heart center is closed in another, including the amount of heart center closure. If you suspect that your heart center is closed to some degree, you may be able to sense how much it is. However, since it is harder to work with yourself with these subjective feelings, if you experience any of the effects noted here, know that it is, and do the crystal work to work with yourself.

Whenever someone presents with the emotional issues discussed above, know that their heart center is closed to some extent, and you can use the following crystals and stones in your emotional healing kit to start carefully opening it. You can also use the heart-centered crystals as a general tonic and emotional "tune-up." If nothing else, it will feel great for yourself and for any other person you work with. Here are the most important crystals for heart opening to have in your emotional healing kit.

ROSE QUARTZ

Other than your clear quartz crystal used to change the emotional vibratory patterns that were just described, the most important crystal to have in your emotional healing kit is rose quartz. There is likely no better crystal or stone to work with the heart. You should have one larger

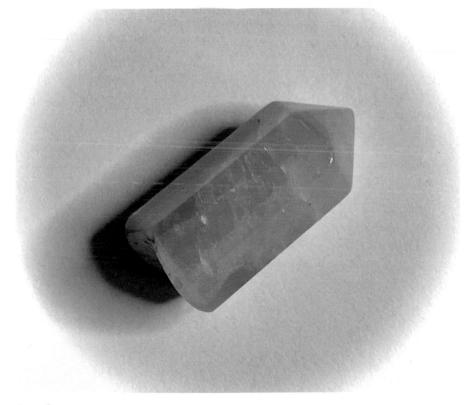

Rose Quartz

piece for placement on the heart center, two medium sizes to hold in the hands, and eight smaller ones to surround the body.

This soft pink stone normally comes in chunks, rarely in crystal form. Generally, if you have a rose quartz shaped like the typical crystal, it has been cut and polished. Either the raw chunk of rose quartz, a tumbled rose quartz, or a cut and polished one can be used. A cut and polished six-sided crystal-shaped rose quartz, however, can be easily used to pull out, send in, or otherwise manipulate emotional vibratory patterns. Although emotional upset can manifest in many parts of your body, the most important place that emotions reside is in your heart center in the middle of your chest. This is true of both positive and negative emotions. We feel all emotions in our heart center. The use of a rose quartz on the heart center will enable the work with all emotions. It is soft and gentle, yet powerful. You can also place a rose quartz anywhere on the body where there is shielding or resistance that needs softening. You can surround the body with rose quartz to help with all emotional healing.

PINK TOURMALINE

Pink tourmaline is a secondary pink crystal that can be used to stimulate or open the heart center. Pink tourmaline has a little more "fire" to it than the rose quartz and thus is not quite as gentle. Where rose quartz envelops in a sense of safety and acceptance when it is used, pink tourmaline can be used when stronger measures are needed. Instead of a sense of enveloping, pink tourmaline is more forceful. When there is great resistance to having the heart center opened or even to feel difficult emotions, this is a great crystal to use. Imagine its bright and strong pink light entering the heart center and easily penetrating through walls of resistance. After penetrating the walls of the heart, it works well to then surround the heart center with a ring of rose quartz. This, then, is probably the second most valuable crystal to have in your emotional healing

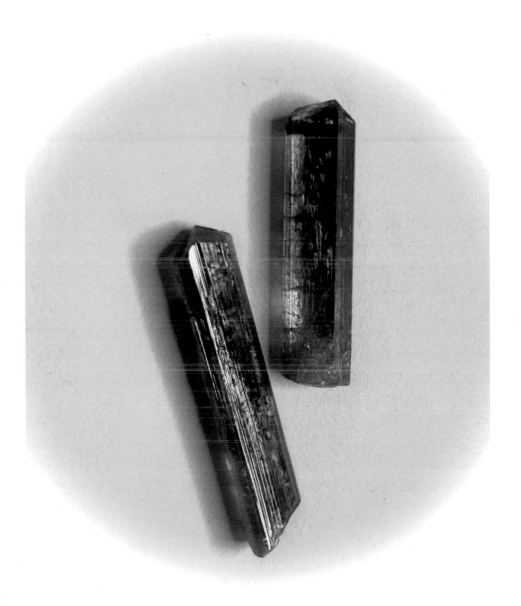

Pink Tourmaline

kit. It is good to have one larger pink tourmaline and four smaller ones to surround the heart center or place on the four sides of the body.

PINK CALCITE

This is a stone that is especially good for developing empathy, and it allows you to attune to the energy fields around you instead of fearfully resisting them. It helps bring a soft, mothering, feminine quality to your emotional healing work that works especially well with trauma. It is good to have one larger pink calcite for placement on the heart center, two others to hold in the hands, and four smaller ones to surround the heart center. You may also want to have four more smaller pink calcites to place around the body.

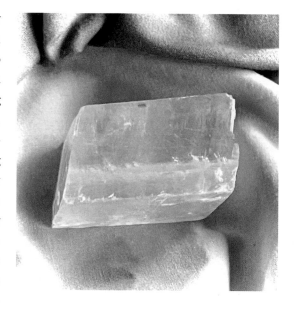

Vibrationally, pink calcite is like being hugged in the arms of the mother, so it is excellent for working with emotional issues associated with the person's mother, their own mothering, and mothering energy in general. Of course, all mothering issues will likely stem back to rejection or early experiences with the person's mother.

If the person you are working with has deep-seated emotional issues with their mother, the energy of pink calcite may be difficult to accept at first, especially if you let them know that this is a crystal associated with mothering. As the mothering energy approaches their heart, they may erupt in hatred or sadness and reject this stone's energy. If so, place a rose quartz on their heart center as you ask the other person if they are willing to let you know what they are feeling in this present moment. (If they cannot come up with a feeling, ask them to imagine a feeling that they might be having.) As they reveal the feeling, place a pink calcite above the heart center. Once this is done, ask if they would be willing to reveal another feeling, especially one about their mother. Again, if they cannot reveal a feeling about their mother, ask if they are willing to imagine a feeling and reveal that. Let them know that it is okay to have hostile or other "bad" feelings about their mother, that you will not be surprised or put off by these. Place another pink calcite below the heart center. Continue with the revelation about these feelings and place a pink calcite on each side of the heart center to eventually surround it. It is not important for the other (or yourself) to understand or reason *why* they have these feelings. The reason is not important at this point, only that they have them. Once you feel you are finished and the pink calcite surrounds the heart center, use the long, deep, breathing technique in and out of the heart, to soften the heart, allowing all of these feelings to exist rather than hiding or resisting them. Besides helping heal deep mother wounding, this process will help bring a sense of compassion for themselves and others.

PINK CORAL, PINK PEARL, OR PINK SHELL

All corals, pearls, shells, and mother of pearl are formed in the ocean or fresh water and carry the essence of this water energy. Water is seemingly gentle, and yet its gentleness should never be confused with lack of power. Water can cut or wear its way through everything. It can also oppose enormous amounts of strength—the strength of boulders, mountains, and all forms of seemingly stable and immovable land masses. Water also brings life that all beings depend on. Without water, life ends.

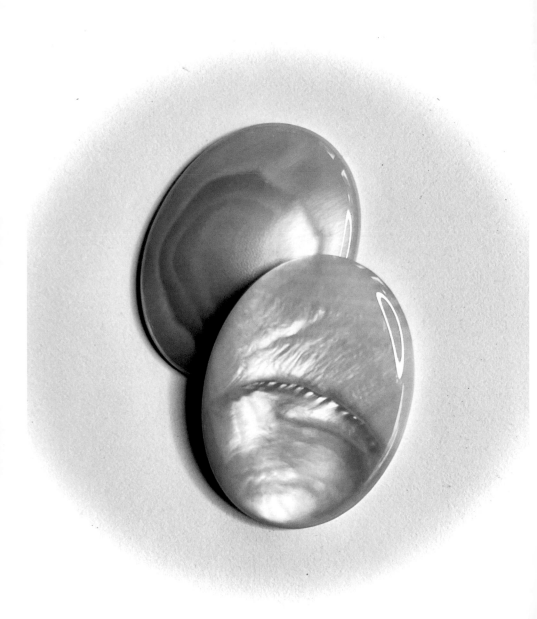

Pink Shell

Though water has strength, it is not rigid but is flexible, mutable, and ever-fluctuating.

Emotions have long been associated with water because of their ever-changing, fluid nature and their mutability. Emotions can seem dark and mysterious, yet pink coral, pearl, or mother of pearl remind us that they also contain light. Like emotions, water can also seem soft and yielding as well as terrifying if you lose yourself in its grip.

These pink forms of shell and pearl help bring love and acceptance to counter the fearful emotions that may hold you in their grip. Though not stones, but growths of protective nacre in the bodies of shell, these pink pearls and corals are excellent in helping release emotional fear and rigidity. They can easily be used to help you accept emotional changes as you go through the transformation of emotional healing work.

Pink mother of pearl, shell, pearl, and coral are beautiful with their iridescence, bringing rainbows of hope and reminding us of the healthiness of tears. As you hold these pink shells on your heart center, or on areas of your body in which emotions are held and stuck, you can remind yourself and others that it is okay to cry, that emotional change can be positive and good, and that outward shows of emotion do not make you weak. Since negative emotions are very often defensive in nature, keeping you from experiencing deep pain, it can be felt that letting them lose will be dangerous and self-destructive. Pink mother-of-pearl, pink pearl, or pink coral can be used to remind you that not only can negative emotions change, but as they change from negative to positive, you become stronger. They are very good, then, for building trust in and allowing the process of emotional change and positive transformation.

Water is also associated with the intuitive moon energy. These pink pearls and corals can be used to help open the intuitive powers that will help bring insight to the overall healing process. Their use will also help you access the increased insight to reach deep within your emotional state to reveal its truth and message that you can then use in your emotional healing.

These pink pearls and corals are very good when surrounding the crystals on the heart center to help accept the truth of your emotions and help you feel safe as they shift. As mentioned earlier, it works very well to place one or more of these on any area of the body in which negative emotions are held to help them become more flexible and allowing of change. It is good to have eight smaller pieces of pink coral, pearl, or mother of pearl. That way you will have enough to use in any situation or to surround the entire body.

> **ALLOWING YOUR EMOTIONS TO POSITIVELY FLOURISH BRINGS YOU STRENGTH.**

Protection and Grounding Crystals and Stones

The following are some protection and grounding crystals and stones that you should have in your emotional healing kit. Each crystal or stone is presented with a discussion of its properties and how it is used. Following that are some further discussions about personal boundaries, grounding, and fear, their typical manifestations, and ways to work with them.

BLACK TOURMALINE

Black tourmaline is known as a crystal that carries the strongest protective powers. Formed of iron and manganese, it has vast charging, grounding, and magnetic powers. Besides providing you a sense of emotional protection, it is known as a crystal that can be used to clear yourself

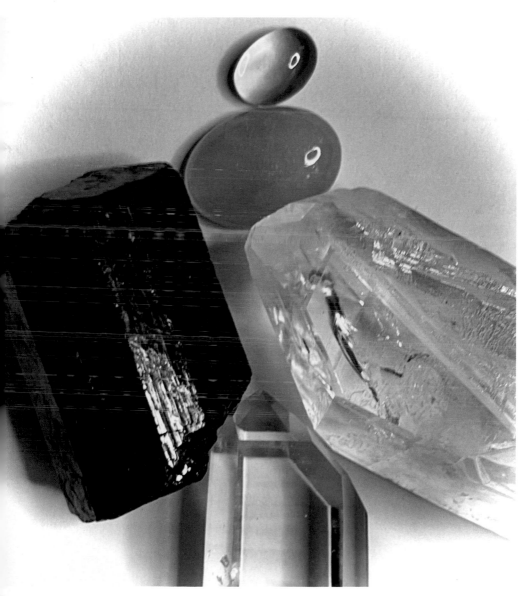

Protection and Grounding Crystals

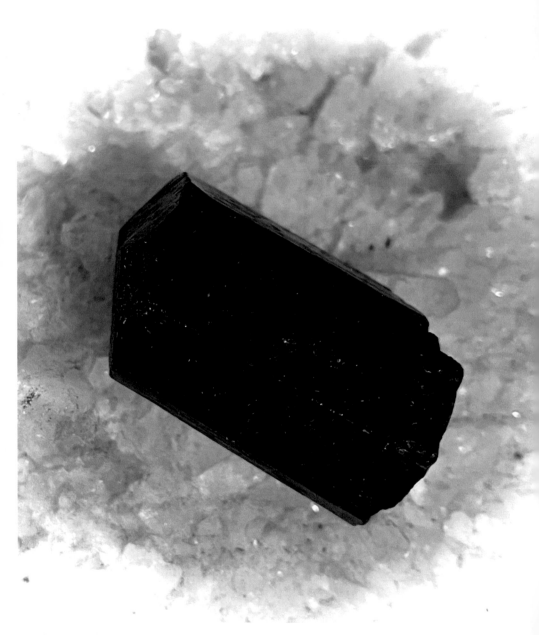

Black Tourmaline Crystal

of all toxic energies as well as of the toxic energies from other people. A strong grounding force, it helps keep you connected to the strength of the earth so that you can use its strengthening life-force energy for your own power. It is known to help bring you the self-confidence that springs from your sense of your own potency. It will help strengthen your protective aura and repel negative or dark energies coming your way. It can help cut through any anxiety that you may have, protect you from the negative energies of others, combat stressful feelings, and help foster a sense of personal power. This is a must-have for your emotional healing kit.

You should have at least one larger piece of black tourmaline. A piece that is approximately 2 inches by 1.5 inches is good to have. Even better is a piece up to 3 inches by 2 inches. The piece does not have to be terminated since you are not going to be directing subtle energy as much as using it to empower. You should also have at least four smaller pieces to surround the body when needed or to hold an equal sized piece in each hand.

BLACK ONYX

Black onyx, a variation of chalcedony, a silicate mineral, is also an excellent stone to use for protection. Where it is sometimes felt that black tourmaline can provide protection that is too impermeable, too strong, or harsh as to be imbalanced with the other subtle emotional energies, black onyx can be a good alternative. Where black tourmaline can feel harsh and repelling, black onyx feels softer and yielding in its protective powers. It can also feel much more calming than black tourmaline, so it is good to use this when you are working with grief and anxiety and need the balance between being grounded and protected yet open and yielding.

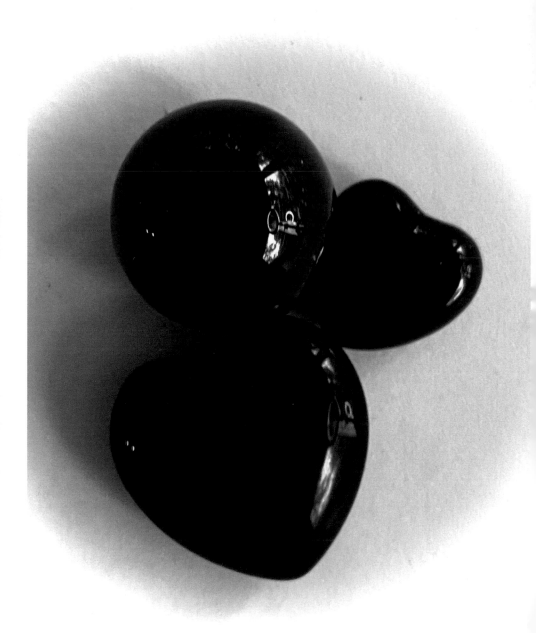

Black Onyx

Place black onyx beneath the bottoms of each foot, beneath each knee, and slightly beneath your tailbone, and it will help connect you with the earth's energies to bring you physical and emotional strength that is calm and centered. It is used to clear and help process issues associated with worry and anger. It is known to help clear up mental unclarity when there is confusion and doubt, helping bring clarity and calm to the associated emotional states. It is said that wearing it will not only bring you a sense of strength and protection, but it will help prevent the draining of your personal energy. In that way, it is very good to have with you when you are around people who tend to be overpowering, overbearing, demanding, or overly needy.

Whether working with protection or grounding, a piece of black onyx beneath each foot or the base of the spine will work well. When you feel that it is too strong to use black tourmaline, you can use black onyx to surround the body to create a protective aura. It can be worn with rose quartz and citrine instead of black tourmaline if more gentleness is needed. It is good to have at least four pieces of equal-sized black onyx in your emotional healing kit.

BLACK AGATE

Black agate and black onyx look so similar that it is sometimes hard to tell them apart. Not only are they both composed of chalcedony and quartz, but they also have similar effects when you use them with emotional healing. Black agate will also provide a gentler form of protective feeling just like black onyx. Like black onyx, it can be used to help establish a strengthening and protective energetic aura around the body to bring calm, focus, emotional strength, and a sense of personal potency. Since they are so similar, it is hard to tell which of these stones to use. The answer is to use the one that you are most drawn to at the moment of your emotional healing. It is said, however, that black agate is a better

Black Agate

stone for grief work, to relax your mind, and limit overthinking. Less overthinking will often help calm emotional turmoil so that your feelings become more stable. Like black onyx, it provides helpful vibrations that help bring you stamina and self-confidence.

Though it is not necessary to have both black onyx and black agate, it is useful, however, to have both. Sometimes, as you focus on the emotional healing to be done, you may realize that black agate is a better crystal to use in the moment, that its energy is "smoother," calmer, and more enveloping than onyx would be. It is recommended that you have both black agate and black onyx in your emotional healing kit. Just like black onyx, have four equal-sized pieces. Or you may have four smaller pieces of black agate to work along with the four black onyx. Basically, this is to give you more options. Be careful when you choose your black agate because much of it is dyed. Be sure to get the natural agate.

SMOKY QUARTZ

Smoky quartz is another valuable crystal for your emotional healing kit. It is both protective and grounding yet so gentle that it is exceptionally easy to accept for anyone who might be resistant to either. Perhaps, for example, someone is emotionally attached to always having to feel "up" or highly energetic and, as a result, will then resist any grounding. Anyone addicted to speed, speedy thoughts, lightning quick emotional swings, constant excitement, or exaggeration will certainly resist you doing anything to impede, slow down, or stop this over-excited energy. Though this energy may feel good, it can be physically, mentally, and certainly emotionally draining and thus quite harmful. Not only that, but by being constantly "up," they avoid experiencing any emotional pain hidden beneath. Constant emotional excitement avoids sadness, depression, despair, emptiness, and other such feelings.

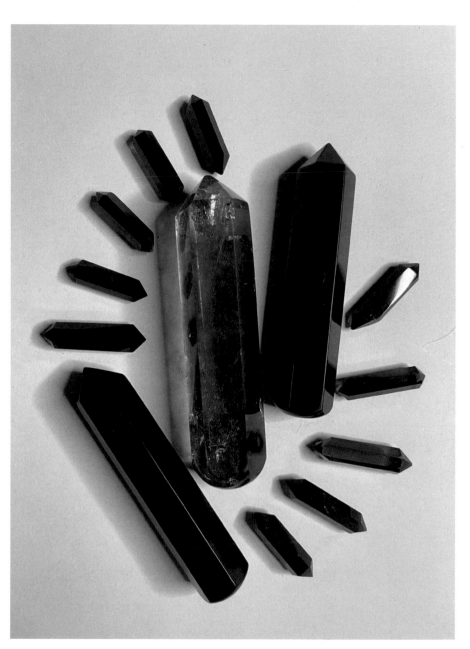

Smoky Quartz

When confronted with this emotional behavior in your sessions, in order to be able to treat the underlying real feelings being repressed or avoided, you need to slow them down. If they are going to resist such slowing, it works best to use the gentler approach of smoky quartz. Smokey quartz is like using a parachute to gently float down to the ground rather than plunging, Floating is easy, gentle, relaxing, while plunging is frightening. Smoky quartz is a soft energy that envelops you in its grounding and protection that is almost impossible to resist since it feels so good.

Don't mistake gentleness with weakness, however. Smoky quartz energy is strong, just quietly so. The same applies with its protective abilities. It will provide a protective aura that is soft and yielding, but at the same time leaves appropriate vulnerability intact. Compared with black tourmaline, onyx, or agate, smoky quartz is more heartful. It is very good for shielding the heart center when needed.

You can use smoky quartz beneath the feet or underneath the tailbone, surround the body, or hold a piece in each hand. You, as the healer, can also hold a single terminated larger piece of smoky quartz in your right hand to raise, lower, remove, or otherwise transform someone's energy in a way that will be more gentle and subtle than using a clear quartz. In your emotional healing kit, it is good to have one larger 3-inch by 1.5-inch single-terminated smoky quartz for active energy manipulation work. Then have about ten smaller single- or double-terminated smoky quartz crystals that are at least 1.5 inches in height.

BOUNDARIES AND EMOTIONAL PROJECTION

When you are doing emotional healing work for another, it is very hard not to energetically absorb their emotions and then feel as if they are your own. This process is amplified if the other person is projecting their emotional state onto you. Emotional projection, as was explained earlier in this book, is when the other person is afraid of, or for some reason, doesn't want to acknowledge and experience that certain difficult or painful emotions belong to them. Rather than face these difficult emotions as they arise, they experience other people as having these emotions. If the person you are working with tends to project their emotional states onto you, it is quite likely that they are doing this in their everyday life as well, experiencing other people as acting or feeling ways toward them that they actually feel within themselves. If the other person tends to project their feelings like this, they will most likely do this to you in your emotional healing session with them.

This dynamic can be very hard to work with during your session because the healing work requires you to leave yourself open and receptive so that you can feel and intuit the other's emotional processes. You can't effectively work with them otherwise. Because of this, it is even harder to distinguish emotions that arise within the other person from those that arise within yourself.

Since emotional projection is a dynamic that you will face often in your emotional healing sessions, it is necessary to know how to work with it, how to distinguish between the other's feelings and your own, and how to protect yourself with appropriate boundaries. The main thing you will need to learn is how to protect yourself from assimilating the other's emotions as your own while remaining aware and open enough to do the work. This can be a delicate balance. If you are too protected, you will never be able to know and penetrate deeply enough into someone's emotional state. If you are not protected enough, you will absorb so much of their emotional state yourself that you will lack the perspective to do the healing work.

PERSONAL BOUNDARIES

The other thing you will probably encounter during your emotional healing work is people who do not know how to establish and maintain

The Ultimate Guide to Emotional Healing with Crystals & Stones

their own personal boundaries, who let people walk all over them and violate their own personal integrity. Though based in fear or a lack of their own sense of self-worth, they usually rationalize this mistreatment in a more positive way, or at least in a way that makes it seem more emotionally tolerable. They may feel as if they are a better person if they don't react negatively to this mistreatment, for example. They tend to attract other people who routinely physically, mentally, or emotionally mistreat them, particularly in close relationships. Belittling, gaslighting, the silent treatment, constantly raging, threats, frequent criticism, and other such dynamics are some of the typical forms of emotional abuse they endure. Generally, this emotional abuse starts with only occasional occurrences, so that the person gradually gets used to it. By the time it magnifies, as it usually does, the person feels trapped. Or they have been so emotionally battered that they lack the internal fortitude or sense of self-worth that it would take to consciously recognize the abuse or change the dynamic. To handle this emotional abuse, the person will often excuse the other, saying, "It isn't their fault," or "They didn't mean it," "I know they love me anyway," "It is just their nature." In extreme cases, the denial is so strong that they refuse to even consciously understand that it is happening because it feels like their own basic physical or emotional survival is at stake to acknowledge it.

The emotional reactions to this sort of emotional abuse usually involve some sort of repression of their natural reactions to retain the possibility of love that the abuser represents. These emotional reactions vary from denial and "fake happiness," repressed anger and outrage, despair and depression, and other such denial mechanisms. In short, this emotionally damaged person represses their own feelings to contain and handle the emotional abuse.

The feelings that result from emotional abuse can be of recent origin or originate from the past or early childhood. Someone in an emotionally abusive situation is often repeating an emotional pattern learned in early childhood, learning this abusive behavior to be an expression of love if an earlier parent or childhood primary caretaker treated them this way. Either way, this core emotional wounding needs to be treated layer by layer to be healed. Your work as an emotional healer is to change the unhealthy emotional reaction to one that is healthy and appropriate and to bring personal empowerment.

During the emotional healing, you may find yourself experiencing your own strong feelings in reaction. If so, you need to establish some boundaries and abilities to let these feelings pass so you can concentrate on the other person rather than yourself. You also don't want to project your own feelings onto another. This doesn't mean that you can't model appropriate emotional reactions from time to time, as this is often a good way to work within a session. You should be careful, however, that you don't make the emotional session about you, but instead, keep it firmly focused on the other.

HOW TO SET BOUNDARIES WITH CRYSTALS AND STONES

During an emotional healing session, you can use your crystals and stones in two ways: The first is to help establish your own personal boundaries that are firm, yet permeable, which allow you to feel the other person's emotions while protecting your own vulnerability. The second is to use your crystals and stones to help the other establish and maintain their own personal boundaries, working with them to recognize what boundaries are appropriate, effective, and useful. Here are some techniques that you can use:

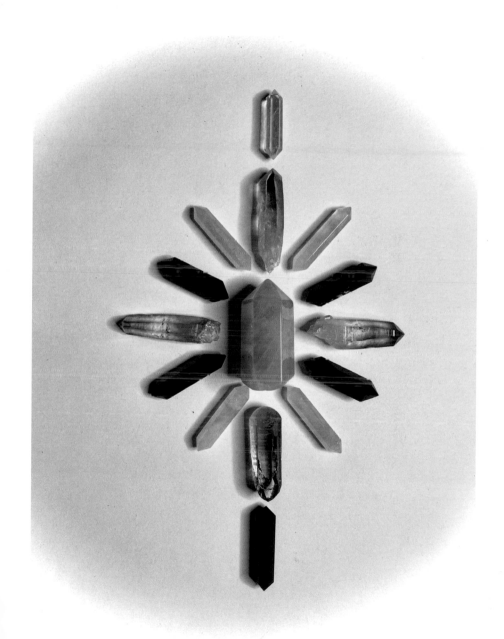

Crystal Layout for Setting Personal Boundaries When Guiding a Healing Session

SETTING YOUR OWN BOUNDARIES DURING A SESSION

1. Before starting the session, wear a clear crystal over your heart chakra with the intention that this crystal helps you shield your heart from absorbing other's emotions while it still remains open and empathetic.

2. Sit in a chair opposite the other person. Have them also sit in a chair facing you. Place a smoky quartz or black tourmaline beneath you. Visualize that this crystal protects you from any negativity in any form. Imagine that any negative emotions, projections, or communications from the other are deflected from your body, mind, and spirit to flow into the earth where they are positively transmuted.

3. Surround your body with alternating amethyst, black tourmaline, or smoky quartz and rose quartz while visualizing that you are enveloped within an orb of protective, loving, and healing light that brings you deep awareness.

4. Surround the other person's body with the same crystals to help them in their process.

5. Hold an amethyst in each of your hands, the tip of the left-hand crystal pointing inward and the tip of the right-hand crystal pointing outward. Hold the intention that all communications from the other be received with wisdom and deep understanding and that all communications from you are wise, appropriate, and healing.

6. During the emotional healing session, listen completely to the other without interruption or judgment so that they feel heard and accepted.

7. Any time you feel any negative feeling within you, ask yourself if it is originating from you or the other. If it is originating from you in reaction to what you are hearing, release the feeling. Imagine that it flows into the earth beneath you where it is positively transformed. If it is originating from the other's projection toward you, instead

The Ultimate Guide to Emotional Healing with Crystals & Stones

of accepting it into you, imagine that it is deflected by your aura of protection to flow into the earth where it is positively transmuted. If the negative feeling is one that you are empathically absorbing from the other, again, let it flow from you into the earth.

8. As the person speaks, let them know what you understand about the way they are feeling, asking if this is their experience. Let them know what you are feeling in response without blaming them for these feelings. Let them know that you are sending any painful or negative feelings into the earth to be transformed. Ask them if they would also like to do the same, releasing the painful feeling to be transformed into the earth.

9. If they are willing, begin to use your crystals to remove and transform the negative or painful feelings, drawing them out and sending them into the earth.

10. At no time accept any negative feeling into yourself as you continue this process.

11. When you are through, be sure to clear the crystals, yourself, the other, and the surrounding environment.

HELPING THE OTHER TO ESTABLISH HEALTHY BOUNDARIES

Helping another set up healthy boundaries against emotional mistreatment can be a long process that takes many sessions as they become self-empowered, gain a sense of their own worthiness, and learn self-respect. As you work with them in your emotional healing sessions to heal the deep emotional wounding that caused the emotional damage and lack of self-worth, personal boundaries will begin to appear as you facilitate this process.

(Continued on next page)

You can use your crystals in your emotional healing sessions to help them start to establish a sense of self boundary and protection. Here is a good method:

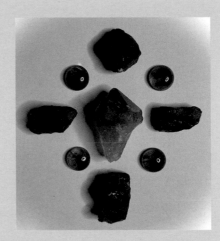

1. Have the person you are working with sit in a chair opposite you. Make sure the distance is one in which you are engaged without being threatening. Usually about 4 to 5 feet is a good distance.

2. Surround the person in a ring of alternating amethyst and black crystals like black tourmaline, black agate, or obsidian. Have them hold a black crystal or stone in each hand. If they are terminated, point the tips outward.

3. Have the person wear an amethyst on their heart chakra so that their heart can remain open yet be protected with the insight to know what to take in or not.

4. Have the person visualize that they are surrounded in a protective aura of personal strength in which no negative communications or feelings will harm them. Have them visualize that any such negativity will either be deflected or be released by them into the healing earth.

5. Have the person silently repeat to themselves, "I am strong. I am worthy. I am free to be me. It is okay to say no."

6. Have the person next visualize that any negative communication or any negative judgment from another, or any negative self-judgment, is repelled rather than received and then released into the earth where it is positively transmuted.

7. After or between sessions, have the person wear or carry an amethyst and a black tourmaline or other black crystal with them every day outside the session, visualizing that a protective black and amethyst aura of light surrounds them. Any time that they experience a negative self-judgment or negativity from another, imagine that it is deflected and sent into the earth. Have them continue to repeat the affirmations in step 5.

> A BOUNDARY IS UNHEALTHY WHEN IT STEMS FROM FEAR AND
> HOLDS YOU FROM LOVE AND ACCEPTANCE.
> A BOUNDARY IS HEALTHY WHEN IT SPRINGS FROM SELF-RESPECT
> AND ALLOWS YOU TO BE TRUE TO YOURSELF.

GROUNDING

It is always tempting to think that the "higher" you feel, the better you will be. This, however, is quite untrue. What you need is balance. If you think of a tree, the branches cannot grow high into the sky until the roots are sunk deep into the earth. Well-established roots bring growth. Likewise, to open to happiness, joy, inspiration, and other qualities of the heart and upper energy centers of expanded awareness, you need to also to feel secure, safe, and "well rooted" with the sense of strength that comes from your lower energy centers being well connected to the earth. This is known as being grounded.

During your emotional healing sessions with your crystals and stones, both you and the person you are working with need to feel the security and balance of being grounded. This is especially true if you or they are overwhelmed or experiencing anxiety, fear, extreme nervousness, or any other intense emotional state. If you feel your jaw tightening, your forehead clenching, your teeth chattering, your body shaking, your shoulders up around your ears, your hands clenching, your breathing shallow and fast, or your body feeling tense, the antidote is to get grounded. If you or the person you are working with can't stop talking or are chattering uncontrollably without anyone getting a word in edgewise, it is good to stop, take some deep breaths, and get grounded and feel your connection with the earth. This will help you or the other person completely relax, breathe deeply, get centered, and find emotional calm.

You can use your earth-toned, gray, or black crystals and stones to help you get grounded. This should be done before every session along with getting centered. Here is a technique you can use to get grounded:

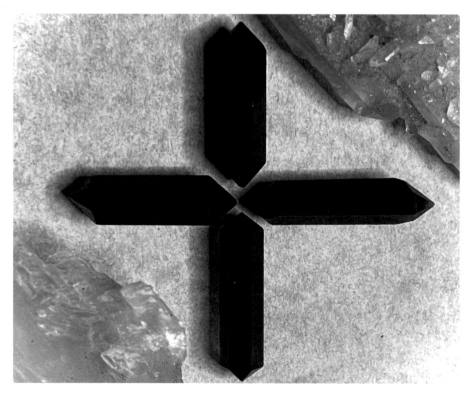

Dark Smoky Quartz for Grounding

The Ultimate Guide to Emotional Healing with Crystals & Stones

CRYSTAL GROUNDING TECHNIQUE

1. Standing or sitting upright, surround yourself with four black crystals or stones, or four smoky quartzes, one in front of you, one behind you, and one at each side of your body. (You can also do this lying down on your back.)

2. Hold a smoky quartz in each hand with its tip pointing down into the earth.

3. Inhale deeply, imagining that your breath enters through your heart center in the middle of your chest. Exhale, imagining your breath flowing down through your body to exit from the bottoms of your feet. As you do this, relax your jaw and head, shoulders, chest, stomach, the small of your back, your thighs, the back of your knees, and your calves. Bend your knees slightly. Feel your connection to the earth (or floor) through the bottoms of your feet.

4. Each time you exhale, feel as if you have streams of earthen light flowing deeper and deeper into the earth from the bottoms of your feet. Your body may be heavier and more solid as you do this.

5. Imagine that you also have earthen-colored beams of light flowing from your fingertips into the earth with each out-breath. As you do this, relax your shoulders, inside of your elbows, and your arms.

6. If you find your mind wandering, let go of the thoughts and bring your attention back to your breath.

7. Continue this for at least three minutes or until you feel yourself centered, relaxed, and deeply rooted into the earth.

8. When you are through, imagine that your breath now flows in and out of your heart center in the middle of your chest. Sweep downward from head to toe with one of your smoky quartz crystals about 6 inches away from the surface of your body. Also sweep downward from your shoulders, down your arms, and out of your fingertips.

9. Clear your crystals when you are through.

Energizing and Protective Solar Crystals

It is very useful to include some yellow crystals or stones in your emotional healing kit because they can bring the fire quality to your protective efforts. Not only can fire resist or "burn up" any negative energy that comes its way, but it also can charge your protective efforts with energy, making them even more effective. Emotional turmoil is physically, men-

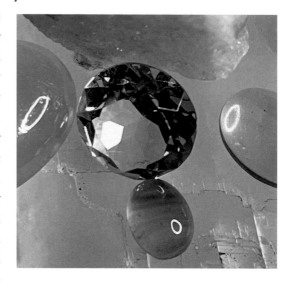

tally, and emotionally exhausting, leaving you feeling drained and incapable of making changes or resisting any negativity coming your way. Empowering yourself with yellow crystals or stones can help.

The following are the yellow-colored crystals that would be useful to have in your emotional healing kit. Though they all have the same basic energizing powers, each one of them is slightly different. The yellow citrine is a strong "blast" of energy compared to the calmer yellow jade or the very soft and gentle yellow calcite. Though you could get by with having only yellow citrine, it is even more useful to couple it with a yellow jade or yellow calcite. That way you can vary the amount of fire energy you add to your protective shield.

YELLOW CITRINE

Like the difference between black tourmaline and black onyx or quartz, yellow citrine has the most direct and powerful fire effect. Instead of a gentle flame, it is like a laser beam. Its fire can penetrate any resistance and overpower any amount of force against it. Its effects are immediate and quick acting. Because of its strength, use it with careful discretion. If the person you are working with is struggling with high anxiety or extreme fear, for example, instead of helping provide a sense of safety and protection, it may do the opposite, providing the fire

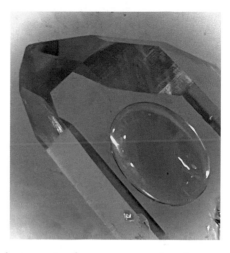

that instead increases these emotional states. In fact, any emotional state that needs calming as well as a sense of protection would probably benefit from the much softer and calmer energy of yellow calcite.

It would be good to have two equal-sized yellow citrines in your emotional healing kit. They don't have to be large because of their power. It is better to have a very clear, diamond-cut citrine rather than a rounded, less clear one. If they are diamond cuts, they only need to be about 0.75 inch in diameter. Place them upside down on the body about 2 inches below and 2 inches above the belly button in line with each other so they feed their energy into the body and the aura. The natural yellow citrine crystals are also good to use. If they have a single termination, you can place them on the body with their tips down or upwards. If their tips are pointing down toward the feet, it tends to be a little more grounding. If they are pointing up, they are more exciting in their energy. If you do use natural citrine crystals, it is best to have them be as clear as possible because they are far more powerful than ones that are cloudy or dull. If clear, they can be almost as strong in their energy as clear diamond-cut citrines. You can also use two round or oval cabochon-cut citrine stones. (This shape has a flat bottom with a domed top.) The energy of this form is a little calmer than the diamond cut or natural yellow citrine crystal, yet still very strong. Be sure when you choose yellow citrines for your emotional healing kit that they are yellow rather than orange or reddish in color.

YELLOW JADE

Yellow jade is not a true jade or jadeite stone. Instead, it is a name for a pale to dark quartz with a yellow coloration. It is sometimes referred to as butter quartz, butter cream quartz, or golden jade. The energy qualities it has are associated with quartz as well as those associated with the yellow color. It is amplifying and energizing. Combined with the fire of the yellow color, it is useful for 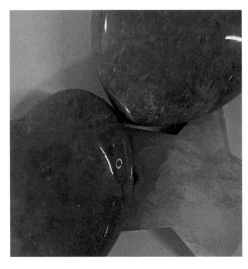 helping build a sense of protection or empowering your black tourmaline, agate, onyx, or smoky quartz protective aura. Not only that, like all yellow crystals, yellow jade can help strengthen any subtle and physical nervous system depletion that usually results from emotional pain and turmoil.

If you choose to have yellow jade in your emotional healing kit, choose ones that are bright yellow as opposed to ones that are more mustard colored. The mustard-colored stones have a lot of earth influence in them so will not provide the fire that will adequately create the sense of protection that you need. Nor will they provide the fire needed to resist or counteract threatening negative energies. Again, be sure that

The Ultimate Guide to Emotional Healing with Crystals & Stones

the yellow jade is natural rather than dyed, which it often is. As with the others, it would be good to have two equal-sized larger round cabochon stones of about 0.75 inch diameter that can be placed both below and above the belly button.

YELLOW CALCITE

Yellow calcite is a great crystal to use when you want to add an extremely gentle, non-threatening fire quality to empower your protective aura. These gentle beings of the crystal world are not only physically soft, but they also provide a sunny, bright, soft yet powerful energizing quality to your protective work. It is to yellow citrine like smoky quartz to black tourmaline. If you want to work very tenderly, soothingly, kindly, and carefully with someone who is highly emotionally overwrought, anxious, combative, or resistant, this is a far better crystal to work with than a bright yellow citrine or yellow jade.

Yellow calcite will help bring a sense of optimism to your emotional healing work. It can bring a sense of hopefulness and a sense of self-confidence. Its softness greatly encourages a sense of cheerful serenity and mental clarity. Its ability to help calm thoughts will help calm the emotions as well, bringing a sense of relief from the pain of emotional chaos, upheaval, and confusion. Its angelic qualities will also help bring a sense of upliftment and relief from any negative experiences of oneself, expanding all negative self-descriptions to those beyond such a limited sense of personal value and worth.

It is good to have at least four yellow calcite crystals in your emotional healing kit that are at least 2 inches in height and width. They can be used below and beneath the belly button to augment your protection aura. They can be used to surround the body to help bring strength to the physical body, the subtle and physical nervous system, and channel in the fire element to combat emotional states that are too cool, like

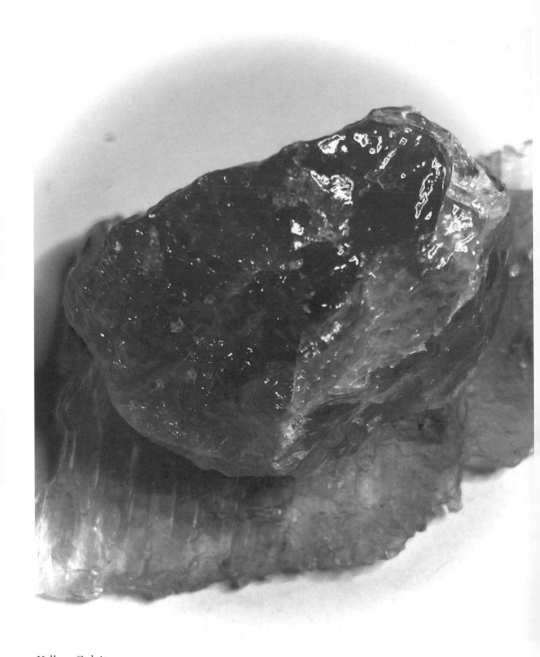

Yellow Calcite

depression and apathy. Four yellow calcites that surround the rose quartz on your heart center are a good way to uplift states of grief, depression, despair, and other such emotions.

WORKING WITH FEAR

Yellow crystals combined with gold tiger eye or black crystals are excellent for working with fear. They can be used to protect against the feelings of fear as well as bring a sense of protection and personal power.

Fear can both help and harm us. Healthy fear helps us identify and avoid threats to our safety. It can be a healthy response to specific objects or situations that would cause us physical, mental, or emotional danger. It is a healthy response, for example, if we are confronted with a snake, walk by a dark alleyway late at night, are approached by a vicious or threatening person, or find ourselves in a violent or menacing situation. It alerts us to the presence of danger and the threat of harm. Stimulating our flight or fight response brings us the energy to react accordingly to real threats. In this way, fear is helpful.

Since the emotional response to fear involves some of the same chemical reactions in our brain as positive emotions like excitement and happiness, some people may have a positive response to fear and may even do things to induce this, such as creating scary, risky, or thrill-seeking situations for themselves. They can also seek out people or relationships that scare them or seem risky. In this case, fear can be perceived in a positive way.

Fear can also be unhealthy and counterproductive when it is in response to an *imagined* future or *imagined* dangers. It can lead to emotional distress and emotion disruption when it is too extreme for the situation or out of proportion to the actual threat. It can be experienced as feeling out of control, panicked, having a sense of impending doom, of being overwhelmed or highly anxious. It can also be physically

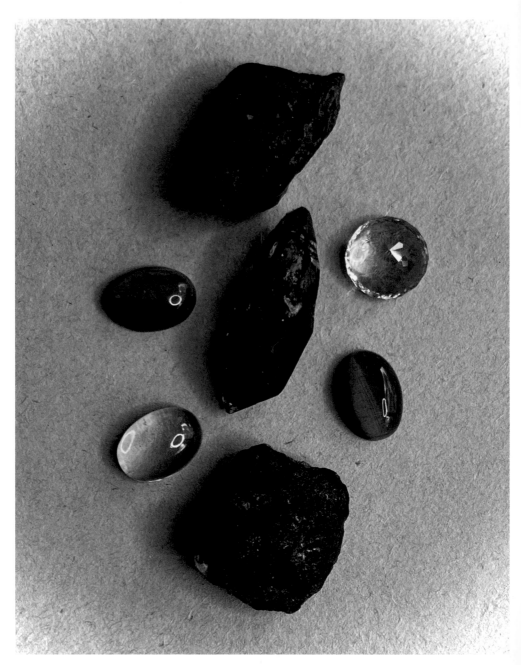

Lava, Black Rutilated Quartz, Citrine, and Gold Tiger Eye

experienced by shaking, nausea, chills, pains in the chest or an upset stomach, a clenched jaw, or overall muscle tightness.

In your emotional healing sessions, you will very likely encounter fear-based emotional reactions to both real and imagined dangers to your well-being and personal safety, or to the well-being and safety of the person you are helping. Whether you are working with your own emotional healing or the healing of another, it is first important to discover if the fear is of a situation or person that really does pose an actual and imminent danger to yourself or the other person. If not, continue your work. If you or the other person are in a dangerous physical situation, or if you or they are with a dangerous person who is a real threat, then you or they need to escape the situation or person right away. Your session, then, needs to focus on how to leave the person or situation.

If you find yourself confronted with deep-seated phobias and other such anxiety disorders in the person you are working with, you will need to work with desensitization techniques. This will help the other person manage the fear response with new coping techniques, with exposure to and confrontation of the fear in a controlled environment, until they realize that they are okay. If you are confronted with this type of phobia or other anxiety disorder in your sessions, however, it is important that you also enlist the help of a trained mental health professional unless you have such training yourself.

In your emotional healing sessions, whether the fear is based on an imaginary future or on past wounds, a good way to work is to explore its dynamics. Every time that fear is felt when imagining a person or event, bring those thoughts back to the present moment. Explore whether that fear is justified based on their current actions or if the fear stems from deeper wounding that magnifies its threat. If you feel fearful of the person with whom you work, end the session immediately and don't be in their presence anymore.

PAY ATTENTION TO FEAR.

IT TELLS YOU SOMETHING IS WRONG.

SHIELDING FROM FEAR

You can use your crystals and stones to create a shield that protects you from what you fear. Feeling protected, you will be better able to work with the fear. You can do this for yourself or another.

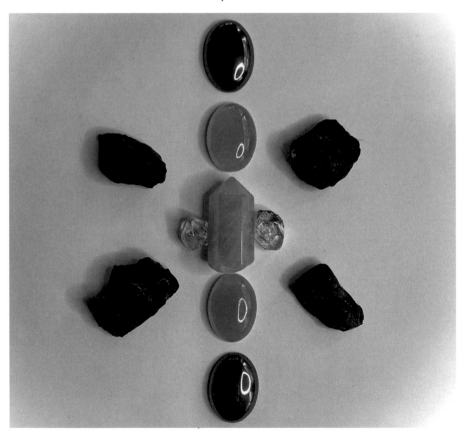

Crystal Layout to Shield from Fear

The Ultimate Guide to Emotional Healing with Crystals & Stones

CRYSTAL TECHNIQUE TO SHIELD AGAINST FEAR

1. Lay flat your back with your legs uncrossed, your arms at your side, and your palms facing upward.
2. Start by surrounding your body with black tourmaline, black onyx, black agate, or other black stones.
3. Place a rose quartz on your heart chakra in the middle of your chest.
4. Place a gold citrine, yellow jade, yellow calcite, or other yellow crystal or stone on your abdomen about 2 inches above your belly button.
5. Place another gold citrine or yellow crystal or stone about 2 inches below your belly button.
6. Hold a single-terminated clear quartz crystal or a double-terminated Herkimer diamond in each hand. If single terminated, point the tips outward.
7. Slow your breathing as you breathe with long, deep breaths. Feel as if these breaths flow in and out of the rose quartz and your heart center. Do this for three minutes or until you feel calm and centered.
8. Imagine that your in-breath flows into your heart center and then out through the yellow crystal on your abdomen. On the next breath, imagine that your breath flows in through the yellow crystal on your abdomen and then out through the other yellow crystal on or below your belly button. On your next breath, imagine that your breath flows in through the yellow crystal below your belly button, out through the bottom of your spine, and out through the bottoms of your feet, connecting you to the strength of the earth. Repeat this entire pattern for at least eleven breath cycles or eleven minutes, feeling yourself growing in power and strength.
9. Shift your breathing so that it seems to flow in and out of your heart center and the rose quartz crystal. With each in-breath, feel as if you are gathering power into yourself. On each out-breath, imagine that

(Continued on next page)

that power flows outward to strengthen your protection aura so that it gets stronger and stronger. Do this for three minutes.

10. When you are through, gather this sense of power and strength to the very center of your being as you continue to breathe in and out of your heart center.

11. Silently repeat to yourself: "I am powerful, protected. I am safe to speak and live my truth."

I AM POWERFUL AND PROTECTED.
I AM SAFE TO SPEAK AND LIVE MY TRUTH.

As you go about your daily life, you can create a shield with your crystals by wearing a neckpiece or pendant with three crystals: a rose quartz, black tourmaline or another black crystal, and a yellow citrine or yellow crystal. They should be of equal size. The rose quartz will help keep your heart open as the black crystal strengthens your protective aura while the yellow crystal brings you the energy to combat the fear and replace the vital energy depletion that fear brings. This way you will be able to remain strong while still also retaining the vulnerability that allows relationships and enhances your ability to hear another's communication.

It is very important to realize that feeling protected and strong doesn't mean that you shouldn't also remain open and vulnerable. The proper balance is to be both permeable and impermeable, both vulnerable and invulnerable, with the wisdom to always know the proper balance between the two, with all people, and in all situations.

As you see, working with fear takes balance. First, you need to listen to the message that fear is telling you. Next, you need to provide yourself a sense of protection from what it is that you fear. Then, when you feel safe, you can face the fear and correct the conditions on which it is based, imaginary or otherwise.

Communication Crystals and Stones

HEALTHY AND UNHEALTHY COMMUNICATION

Good communication fosters mutual understanding, openness, a sense of mutuality and togetherness. Words can bring you together with others or drive you apart, not only by what you say, but by how you say it. In other words, your words can draw people to you or send them running. With healthy communication, you can communicate your wants and needs so that people have a chance to satisfy them. If you can communicate how you feel, then people will feel free to share themselves emotionally with

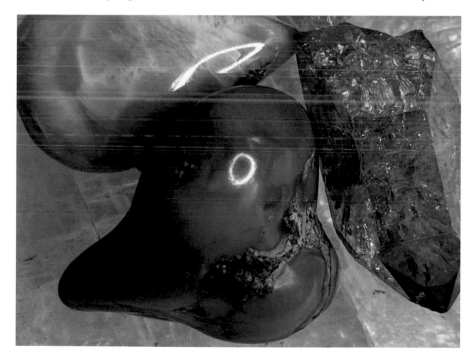

Turquoise, Larimar, and Aqua Aura Communication Crystals

you. Being able to communicate your true feelings will help bring you the understanding and positive emotional response that will create deep and satisfying relationships.

Healthy communication is when you can completely listen to another, letting them express themselves without correcting or judging them. It acknowledges that you understand how they feel and believe, whether you feel or believe the same yourself. It acknowledges that others have the right to be themselves, and that you find them interesting just as they are, that they don't need to be any different than they are.

GOOD COMMUNICATION FOSTERS MUTUAL UNDERSTANDING AND OPENNESS.

Healthy communication also means that you can express yourself freely, that you feel free to be yourself, that you don't have to pretend to be any other way than you are. It reflects the expression of your own sense of value and positive self-worth. When you can communicate with another in a healthy manner, you are able to skillfully express your wants and needs, that you feel deserving of their satisfaction as much as anyone else. Healthy communication is nourishing rather than depleting. It is an expression of openness, compassion, and mutual acceptance, bringing both you and the other a sense of joy and satisfaction. It is the bridge to true companionship. In your work with emotional healing, this is what you want to help the other person, or yourself, achieve.

When communicating with others, it is important to let them know that you care about them. This doesn't mean that you need to tell them that you love or really like them for them to feel this. Instead, it means that your communications should nonverbally convey your care by allowing the other person to share themselves with you, by accepting them as they are, by avoiding shame, blame, or other negative judgments as you speak or otherwise interact. Someone should be able to relax and be themselves with you instead of feeling that you will only care about them if they act or say things you approve of. It should not be important that someone agree with you, only that you both can respect and share different points of view.

In that way, good communication fosters real relationships that help you feel accepted and understood. Much loneliness, sadness, depression, anxiety, shame, and other such negative emotions can be avoided or healed with the use of better communication, the kind that allows people to really know and understand you rather than the kind that keeps you apart.

It is important that your emotional healing sessions model healthy communication. Not only will this help you be more effective in your work, but it also teaches the other person what is good, effective communication and what is not.

UNHEALTHY COMMUNICATION

Unhealthy communication is the opposite. Instead of bringing you together, poor communication skills keep you apart from others. If you don't express yourself, no one will know how you feel, and your emotional needs are likely to remain unfulfilled. If your words are hostile or off-putting, they will drive others away from you. If you talk so much that no one can get a word in edgewise, people will stay away from you, feeling like you don't really want to know and interact with them. If you talk "at" someone, using your words as an emotional barrier instead of a bridge between you, you will forfeit any real connection between you and others. Your relationships will remain shallow and unsatisfying at best.

One of the main reasons people fail to communicate in a way that draws people to them rather than causing them to flee is that the negative ways they feel about themselves are projected outward onto others so that they experience others as, in turn, judging them negatively. By doing that, their experience is that the other person feels that way about them, not that they feel that way themselves. In other words, it is emotionally safer to feel that others have these "bad" feelings rather than owning them yourself. If you have to actually feel these negative feelings yourself rather than avoiding them, it would subconsciously affirm that you are "bad," "unworthy," "shameful," or otherwise deficient. If you feel an inward sense of unworthiness, for example, you will tend to experience others around you as being unworthy of your attention, or never being able to live up to your expectations. If you feel unloved, you may experience others as unloving toward you and respond to them with rejection. In reflection of this emotional projection, words and actions are then consciously or subconsciously used to drive people away before they can hurt you in ways that you think they might. For example, if you don't want to risk the feeling of being unloved like you were in early childhood, you may drive people away with hateful or dismissive words before you possibly risk being unloved or unliked by them. Communications of anger, abruptness, judgment, belittlement, rudeness, disgust, or similar negative emotions are designed to attack and consciously or unconsciously drive people away from you. They may also be designed to keep you in a superior position if you feel inferior to people—again, a feeling that most likely stems from early childhood wounding.

These negative communications do not have to be verbal. They can also be accomplished with actions. Turning your back on someone, for example, communicates your anger or disgust without having to even say the words. Ignoring someone lets them know that you consider them unworthy of your attention. Similarly, rolling your eyes when someone says something to you, or sighing like you find their words hopelessly stupid, also communicates quite clearly without saying anything. Of course, hitting, striking out against someone, or doing something to actively hurt someone is its own form of communication that needs no words to be understood. These actions are a form of attack. Whether by design or not, they will keep people away from you.

> ## MOST PEOPLE WANT TO BE UNDERSTOOD. MANY ARE AFRAID
> ## TO BE BECAUSE OF THEIR OWN NEGATIVE SELF-JUDGMENT.

WORKING WITH COMMUNICATION IN YOUR EMOTIONAL HEALING SESSION

You will find both positive and negative communications toward you in your emotional healing sessions. The deeper you get in your emotional healing work, the more you will be able to peel away the outward emotional layers to reveal what lies beneath. As you do this, quite often the person you are working with will begin to "act out" their deeper, more painful, internal emotional states in reaction to this. As you get closer to this core wounding in your healing efforts, the other person may feel so threatened that they need to drive you away. It is important to know, in this case, that even though they may overtly be trying to drive you away, down deeper, they really don't want to. They want your help. They are just afraid. So, don't let yourself be driven away. If this happens, instead of being offended, angered, or driven off by negative communications, or torrents of words that don't allow you to get close, or the outright silence of no communication at all, it is important to understand from where these communications originate and what purpose they serve. Just know that these are a sign that you must proceed more carefully and tenderly. Again, rather than responding to the acting out, use your intuition, expanded awareness, and careful attention to discover its source. That is where your healing actions should be focused.

This does not mean that you should let the other person be free to mistreat you during the session. Not only does this do you no good, but it is also not helpful for the person you are working with. Instead, name the action and let them know that it is inappropriate for them to say or do this to you. Then use it as a springboard to reveal what the deeper emotional pain is beneath that seemed to necessitate the mistreatment. Ask them to see if they can pay attention to the feelings they are having at this moment. You can have them place a rose quartz on the heart center and a turquoise on their throat center as you ask them to name the feeling and see if they can thoroughly explore it. Where does it seem to be centered in their body? Can they describe any images coming to them? Can they remember any past events in which they had this same feeling? If they can, explore even deeper, asking them if they can remember any other past events or incidences in which they had this same painful feeling. Did they make any decisions about themselves with respect to this pain? If so, what? Go as far back as they are able, resting with the remembrance of each past event, finding if or where it is stored in their body, and asking about any decisions or negative self-judgments they made about this. Between each remembrance, take a few minutes to breathe with long, deep breaths while focusing on their heart center. See if they can release the pain. Once you are through, help them to be centered and grounded and then guide them to release any lingering pain with each out-breath to then relax with their attention concentrated in their heart center. In this way, their mistreatment can be transformed into a powerful emotional healing event.

Again, as with all effective communication, let yourself thoroughly listen without judging them, telling them they are wrong, or that they should feel differently. Let them know through your careful and complete listening that they are understood and accepted as they are.

There are several crystals that can be used during your emotional healing session that will help you with this communication work. These crystals will help you communicate better yourself, to find the words to accurately express what you are feeling, and to find the words to describe the emotional states you are experiencing from the other. They also can be used to help the person you are working with find the words to describe what they are feeling and communicate them effectively. These crystals and stones will help facilitate both verbal and nonverbal communication as well as overall self-expression. They will also help you release any obstructions to communication and any expression blocked anywhere in your body.

TURQUOISE AND TURQUOISE-BLUE CRYSTALS

Turquoise and turquoise-blue crystals like larimar are excellent stones to have in your emotional healing kit. Turquoise is known as being able to

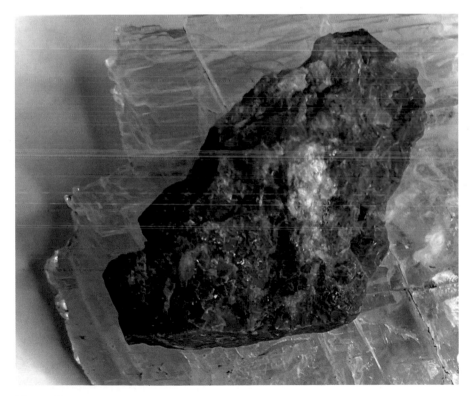

Turquoise

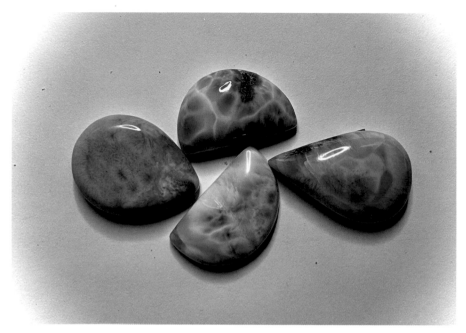

Larimar

absorb negativity in all forms, including negative feelings and communications. All turquoise-blue colored crystals are excellent stones to help release any feelings trapped in the body or mind. They can help release repetitive feelings as well.

There are many ways you can use turquoise to help absorb negativity during your emotional healing session. You can surround your room with a turquoise on every corner, place it around your body, the other's body, have the other person hold a piece in each hand, or hold it yourself, feeling that it will collect any negativity that is expressed or felt during the healing session. Once the session is over, you can clear the negativity by placing it on the earth, imagining the earth absorbing and transmuting the negativity to nurturing energy. Or you can use the smoke method (smudging) to clear out the negativity. If you use the smoke method, imagine that all negativity leaves the turquoise until the stone feels or looks brighter.

You can use larimar to help release negativity by placing it on the body itself. During the emotional healing session, many negative, painful emotions will likely be uncovered. As these emotions are experienced, determine if there is any place in the body where these painful emotions reside or are trapped. Once an area is identified, place the turquoise on that area, and visualize that this emotion releases with every out-breath to flow into the turquoise. Keep doing this until you feel a sense of relief as the emotion lessens or disappears entirely. Once you feel free of the painful emotion, replace it with its opposite. If you like, use a clear quartz crystal in your right hand to send in the opposite feeling.

Yet another technique that you can use is to lie on your back and place a turquoise on the heart center, the belly, the throat, and the lung points between the throat and heart center, one above each nipple. Let yourself feel the painful emotion as completely as you can. With each out-breath, imagine that the turquoise fills with the released painful emotion until it is as completely absorbed as possible. As you do, continue to relax your body. To amplify this effect, you can surround the body with turquoise, as well. As you do this, imagine that your entire aura glows with turquoise blue light. When you are through, place the turquoise stones on the earth and imagine that all the painful emotion flows into the earth to be positively transmuted.

Unless it is a rather superficial emotion, or one that is temporarily passing through your awareness, it is unlikely that this will work to release the problematic emotion or emotional pattern completely. You will probably have to do this many times, or if working with emotional layering, do this for each emotional layer that you uncover.

Turquoise is also known to enhance and facilitate communication, especially when placed on the energy center in the middle of the throat. It is thought to help you find the words to express how you are feeling.

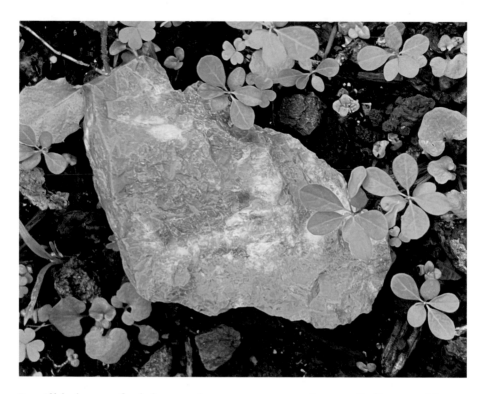

It will help you find the words to express your deepest feelings and inner truth in a way that others can understand clearly. It will help you find the words that are effective at the moment that you speak. It will also tend to help you overcome the fear of communication.

Turquoise is not only helpful for the one being healed but also for the facilitator of the healing. If you are the one helping another heal emotionally, placing or wearing a turquoise on or near your throat energy center will help you find the right words to say that will be most helpful for the healing. It will help you find the words to express what you intuit or "see" with your expanded awareness.

Finally, turquoise radiates the tranquility and peace of endless blue skies, of a translucent and calm sky-blue ocean. When faced with the turmoil of upsetting and painful emotions, this stone will help bring a sense of calm and hopefulness. This tranquil quality helps facilitate clear thinking, also useful for working your way through painful emotions. As it is also known to help silence your inner critic, it also helps to release thoughts of unworthiness, insufficiency, shame, and other such emotional negative valuations of yourself.

It is useful to have at least four equal sizes of turquoise in your emotional healing kit. That way you will have one for each hand, four for the heart, throat, and lung points, or to surround the body or the room in which the healing is taking place.

AQUA AURA

Aqua Aura is created in a vacuum chamber from quartz crystals and pure 24-karat gold vapor. The quartz is heated and then the gold vapor is added to the chamber. The gold atoms then fuse to the crystal's surface, which gives the crystal an iridescent, turquoise, metallic sheen. To get the beautiful clarity that it is known for, only the brightest, clearest, most natural quartz crystal can be used. Aqua aura, besides being beautiful, is a gorgeous turquoise color like a fine aquamarine. Because of the way it is made, it combines the energetic qualities of pure gold and clear quartz. This is combined with the energetic qualities associated with the turquoise color.

Many qualities are attributed to it that are quite useful in your emotional healing sessions. Though it is turquoise colored, it does not have the absorptive qualities associated with a turquoise stone. It does, however, help release whatever is being held or trapped in the body or mind, including painful or repetitive feelings. Not only does it help release them, but you can also then use its angelic qualities to fill these areas with light, peace, upliftment, and joy.

Like turquoise, aqua aura can be used to help bring the ability to express yourself, even your deepest truths. You can find the words to

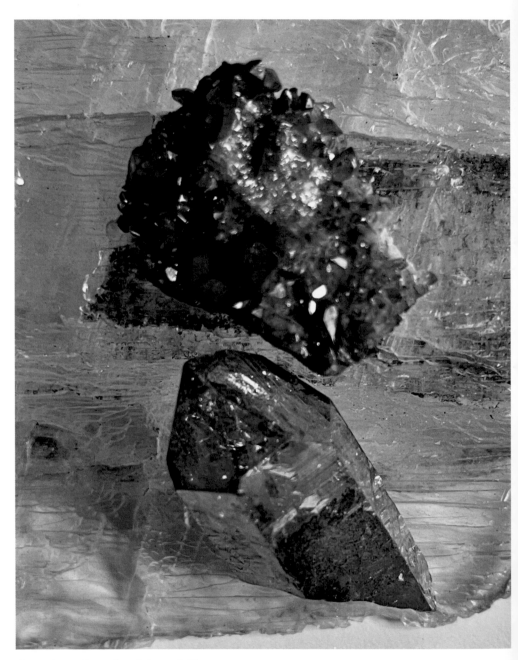

Aqua Aura Crystal and Crystal Cluster

express exactly what you are feeling, even if such feelings seem threatening if they are revealed.

You can use aqua aura to sweep the subtle aura around your physical body to cleanse and heal the physical and mental bodies, as well as the emotional body. Their angelic qualities are used for protection from any negative energy that someone is sending your way. Resonating with your upper energy centers, these angelic crystals are known to help you connect with your higher spiritual self. This connection can be used during your emotional healing sessions to uplift you and to bring higher perspective to help you with your transformative emotional work. Aqua aura will help bring a bright, sunny joyfulness to any session. If your emotions start feeling intolerably "heavy," this crystal will help lighten them. It is especially good to work with to counteract depression, sadness, or despair. Aqua aura will tend to help you speak more truthfully with those to whom you are relating, whether it is someone you have just met or someone with whom you are in a long-term relationship.

It is good to have at least one aqua aura crystal in your emotional healing kit that is approximately 2 inches by 1 inch. This is a good size to use to send the angelic, joyful, and transformative energy into the body and mind of the person you are working with, especially when they are experiencing a painful emotional pattern. To do this, have them hold their hands in front of them, palms upright in a receptive position while you use the aqua aura crystal in your right hand to send in its energy. While this is being done, have the person feel the painful emotion that they would like to be lifted, and imagine that the turquoise blue angelic energy sweeps through their heart and mind, uplifting and transforming the feeling as it does so. Imagine that with every in-breath, this angelic, sky-blue energy fills them with peace and joy.

LARIMAR

Where turquoise is related to earth and sky and aqua aura is related to the sky, larimar is related to water and sky, particularly the water of the ocean. Since it is created from volcanic energy, although it is sky blue, it also brings the energy of fire. Water is mutable, flowing, changeable, and in a constant state of flux. Larimar's qualities that relate to water make it a very good emotional healing stone to help you change anything holding you back emotionally. It will help release rigid beliefs and thought patterns

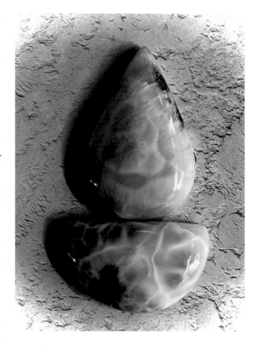

upon which some of your most painful emotional patterns depend. It will help you release old toxic patterns that get in the way of loving and caring relationships and bring the ability to be more spontaneous in your emotional life, allowing you to let go of the ways in which you limit your self-expression. It is also related to sky energies, so is very good to work with releasing old, painful emotional patterns that no longer serve you. It has an expansive quality that can bring you a sense of calm, clarity, and peace. Its relationship to fire and to the sea can help bring emotional balance for those who need inner strength as well as the ability to be emotionally yielding rather than rigid. In that way, it is good for breaking down emotional boundaries that keep us apart from each other. It has the energy of flow and movement, and as such can be used to sweep away anxious, repetitive, debilitating thought patterns that keep us stuck in emotional pain.

Like aqua aura and turquoise, it also helps stimulate the energy center of the throat, the center of communication. As such, like the other two stones, it will help facilitate clear communication and enhance self-expression. Larimar, however, tends to be more soothing in its energy. It is an incredibly calming stone and can help heal all stress-related and toxic emotional patterns. Using larimar in your emotional healing is like bringing a fresh breath of air, a restorative clarity, and a soft stillness to your emotional healing work.

You can select at least one larimar stone for your emotional healing kit to place on your own throat center to help you with your communication during the healing session. Or you can place it on the throat center of the other person you are working to help them express themselves. It is good to use a flat cabochon of any shape because its flat bottom will help it rest nicely in the center of the throat without falling off. If you'd like, you can add two more pieces so that the person you are working with can hold one in each hand to further assist their ability to communicate.

Insight Crystals and Stones

During your emotional healing session, you will often have to intuit what someone is really trying to communicate beyond the words they are saying so that you can help them. Sometimes painful feelings will be quite hard for the other person to tell you about. This is especially true if the communication feels threatening to them, or they think it will make them seem silly, stupid, or somehow a "bad person" in your eyes. They may be lying about how they are feeling so that they keep your respect, or they may not talk at all, just telling you that all is fine while, at the same time, hoping you will see through them and draw the communication out of them. They may be telling you they are perfectly happy; however, with their body closed into itself with their legs crossed and their arms tightly across their middle, you suspect otherwise. If they can't look at you or their eyes look vacant or troubled, for example, that is also a form of communication that may speak louder than their words. Or it may be that you

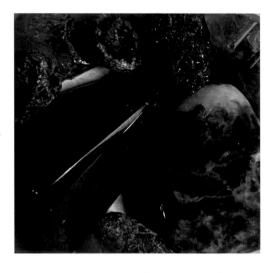

just feel an inner sense of disquiet or unease, so you know something is "off" or that more needs to be said. In cases such as these, you will need to be able to draw upon other ways of knowing and "hearing" other than the verbal.

Intuition is one of the other ways of knowing. It is helpful to learn how to do three things when you listen to the words that someone is saying to you. Besides being able to actively listen to the overt words they are saying, you also need to be able to "read" what their body language is communicating to you and hear what your intuitions and the voice of higher awareness is telling you. These other ways of hearing and knowing are just as valid as logic and, sometimes, may even be more accurate.

Stimulating or opening your upper energy centers will help bring you the ability to "hear" these unspoken, nonverbal communications quite clearly, especially if you learn to trust it. You learn to trust this information that you receive by testing it in the "real world," or in this case, asking the other person if this is what they are *also* trying to say to you, if this is *also* what they meant, or if you are correct in what you are also "hearing" in the words that they aren't saying or in their body language. Notice, instead of negating what they are telling you, or undermining them in any way, you can continue to show your support by enlisting their participation in the search for deeper meaning beneath or beyond their words. After acknowledging that you heard what they said, ask them something like, "I notice that you can't look at me. Is there anything else that you would like to say that you don't feel safe saying?" Or you can ask, "I hear that you are saying that you are not bothered by this feeling that you are having, but I also notice that you are clutching your stomach. Are you also feeling fearful?" Likewise, you can just ask them about what you are "hearing" with your intuitive, expanded awareness, saying something like, "I am intuitively seeing you being chased by something dark and menacing even though you are saying that everything is okay. Are you afraid of someone or something?" If they agree with what else you are "seeing" or "hearing," ask them to elaborate on it, saying something like, "Do you feel like telling me about it?" If so, ask them to elaborate again, asking a question such as, "How so? Tell me about it." If they are not willing to tell you about it, or they tell you that you are wrong, acknowledge that and then ask them to elaborate. You can ask something like, "I hear what you are saying. Can you let me know how I am wrong?" The key is to engage them in a way that encourages them in a nonthreatening manner to open to you further than they have so far. This is an important way to start peeling away the emotional layers that cover up deeper wounding.

You can increase your intuitive abilities by learning to pay more careful attention to subtle feelings in your body that either support or belie the words that you hear. For example, notice if your stomach suddenly feels very slightly nauseous, or if your jaw feels clenched when someone tells you that they are not frightened or that they were never belittled by their parent when they were kids. These subtle feelings may be very slight and hard to discern if you aren't paying attention. Whether a whisper of wind, a minor change in your body temperature, or a slight tightening somewhere in your body, these sensations have their messages for you if you have the ability to intuitively discern them.

Another way to increase your intuitive powers is to stimulate or open your "third eye" energy center in the middle of your forehead between your brows. Sometimes referred to as the "mind's eye," "inner eye," or "eye of consciousness," and associated with the pineal gland and the entire glandular system, this is the center that, when open, is the gate to creativity, intuition, clairvoyance, clairaudience, the ability to "see" auras, the inner realms of spiritual energy, and all forms of perception beyond ordinary sight. When this energy center is enlivened or open, you will be able to easily discern what is being communicated to you beyond the overt words that you hear in and out of the emotional healing sessions that you conduct.

You can use any royal blue crystals and stones to help open this energy center. You can also use a clear crystal or Herkimer diamond. The following are some crystals and stones that are particularly good for opening your third eye and notes on how to use them.

LAPIS LAZULI (LAPIS)

Lapis is perhaps the best crystal or stone to use to open your third eye center. Containing the multiple minerals of lazurite, diopside, calcite, pyrite, and more, its deep, royal blue color, often joined with flecks of gold, is like the star-sprinkled night sky. Representing endless space that extends without limit beyond the bounds of the physical earth, this stone of royalty and courage perfectly matches the color and energy of the third eye energy center. Using lapis powerfully stimulates this center, causing it to vibrate with increasing frequency, and as it does so, it draws the energy of your subtle life force to pierce upward through this powerful portal to expanded awareness into higher realms. As your third eye is thus stimulated and opened, it will bring you clarity, integrity, intuition, wisdom, and the awareness of higher truth.

During your emotional healing sessions, you can place a lapis on your third eye center in the middle of your forehead with a headband. You can also wear lapis earrings that will open your third eye. If you are wanting to pay particular attention to the more subtle communications beyond the words that you are hearing in your session, surround

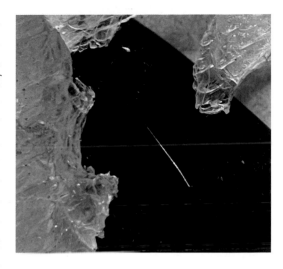

your body with lapis as you sit in your chair, or hold a lapis in your left hand, imagining its energy flowing in through your hand, up your arm, to your throat center, up through your head, and out of your third eye. As you listen to the person you are helping, use your breath to further access the intuitive information you are receiving. Imagine that your in-breath flows in through your heart center in the middle of your chest and out through your third eye in the middle of your forehead. You can do this while you listen. When you are through with the session, be sure to clear the lapis. (After working with lapis during your session, you will likely find that you are increasingly intuitive and aware of expanded realities during your everyday life as well as during the session.)

The person you are working with can also use lapis during the healing session to be able to access deeper truths that may be buried in their subconscious that will help them in their emotional healing process. As the lapis is placed in their left hand, in each hand, or in the middle of their forehead, they may be able to view old childhood events without the blinders of forgetfulness, disassociation, or avoidance. Their ability to use visualization during their healing session will deepen and their inner realms will reveal themselves more completely.

Your emotional healing kits should contain at least one lapis stone that can be placed on the third eye.

BLUE SODALITE

Blue sodalite will also work if you don't have a lapis. They can look very similar, but blue sodalite sometimes has white in it as well as the royal blue or is sometimes darker. It can look almost black. It does not contain the gold flecks that are often within a lapis stone. Sodalite has a feeling of being more earthbound and less anchored to the sky qualities like lapis. If you use sodalite instead of lapis, choose a piece that is royal-blue colored rather than a color tending toward black.

Sodalite will also work to open the third eye, especially if you use a royal-blue colored one. It is thought to help overcome negative thinking, increase mental clarity, and encourage truthfulness as it supports all forms of communication. Because of its earth-bound tendencies, sodalite can be used to inspire confidence and emotional strength. If someone is having trouble retaining their sense of their own reality or letting someone impose their own viewpoints, especially if interacting with a controlling or narcissistic person, sodalite is a good stone to use to avoid becoming emotionally overwhelmed by another. It is a good stone to use when being gaslighted or being told that your experience is wrong in some way. This defense against such emotional intrusion or overwhelm can be further enhanced if you combine a sodalite with one of the black or smoky protection and boundary crystals or stones.

Because of its more earth-bound, protective quality, sometimes you will want to use sodalite instead of lapis in your emotional healing session. For that reason, it is good to have one or two pieces of like-sized tumbled or carved and polished sodalite stones in your kit. They should be at least 1.25 by 1.25 inches in size if they are tumbled. If they are carved into a traditional crystal shape, they should be at least 1.25 inch in height and 0.5 inch in width. Each stone should be small enough to use directly on the third eye in the middle of the forehead, or to be easily held in the left hand or in both hands. If the sodalite is carved into a crystal shape, it is good to use a single terminated with one point. That way you can point the tips in toward the body as you use them to channel their energy inward. If you lay one of these stones on the third eye, point the tip upward toward the top of your head.

BLUE AZURITE

Royal blue azurite is a beautiful, deep blue copper mineral produced by the weathering effects of copper ore deposits. It is known as a stone that can be used to treat disorders and illness in the head and brain, including all forms of headache. It is also known as a good crystal to connect you with the divine energy and act in alignment with your higher self rather than fall prey to your lower impulses. It is believed to be a good crystal to connect you with the desire for justice, peace, and truth. Emotionally, azurite has long been used to help bring a deep understanding of the root of fear, sadness, anger, and other such negative emotions. It is used to help uncover your subconscious beliefs from the past that support painful or uncomfortable emotions and discover whether they are true anymore. In this way, azurite can be a powerful ally in the uncovering and healing of painful emotions that stem from past core wounding. Also used to open and stimulate the third eye, it is even more specifically used to expand awareness past the here and now to work with the past emotional dynamics. It is an especially good crystal to not only use for third eye opening for expanded intuition and other such third eye qualities, but also to work to uncover core emotional wounding and uncover the

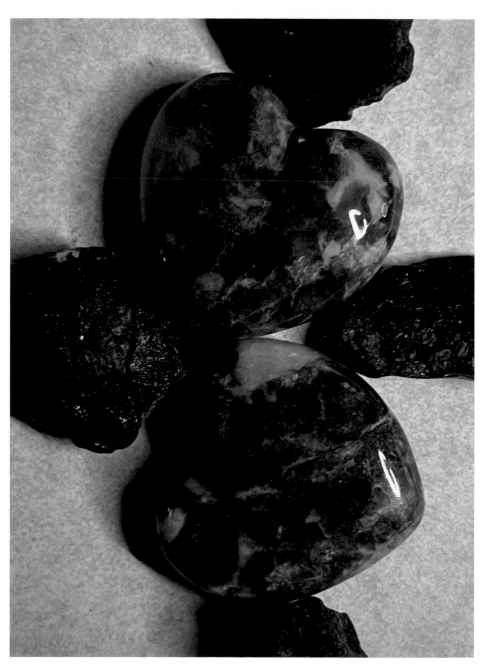

Blue Sodalite with Lava

limiting belief patterns that sustain their effects in the present.

Your emotional healing kits should contain at least one pure royal blue azurite crystal without green, brown, or any other color in it for work with the third eye. Many pieces of azurite are also mixed with green malachite. If you want to work with the heart as well as the expanded insight of

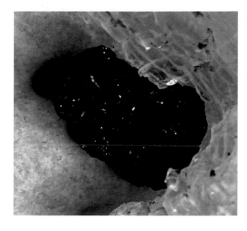

the third eye, an azurite mixed with malachite is a good crystal to have. If your azurite is a vibrant royal blue crystal, you don't need a large one because of its power. A very small one of approximately 0.5 by 0.5 inch is sufficient.

BLUE SAPPHIRE

Sapphires come in many colors: blue, green, yellow, white, violet, red, black, and pink. To open the third eye, the blue sapphire is the one you want to use rather than the other colors. Since they tend to be expensive, people do not often have sapphires in their emotional healing kits, preferring to only use the lapis, sodalite, or azurite. However, you can use a raw sapphire and it will likely have all the power you need to do the third eye opening work.

Blue sapphires are the ones that you should have in order to work with the third eye energies, to increase intuition, and to bring higher forms of insight and knowing. Besides also working to stimulate the throat energy center, blue sapphire is excellent for helping you communicate your inner truth related to your deep, inner self. It is known to help bring you a single-minded focus, a mental/emotional power associated with the third eye. As your third eye is stimulated by this crystal, you will be increasingly aligned with the higher realms and so will easily rise from your enmeshment with lower energy emotions that fail to bring you joy and a sense of well-being. As with the other royal blue stones and crystals, sapphire works well to bring higher insight, increase intuition, stimulate divination, and bring awareness of the higher planes of reality. It is said that using sapphire will help

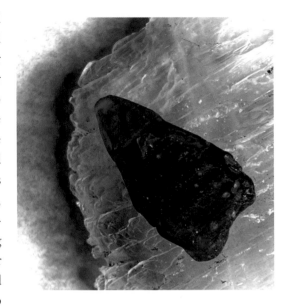

move you from depression and delusion and bring you deep calm. If you meditate with blue sapphire, it will help bring you peace of mind and a deep sense of serenity. Using blue sapphire in your emotional healing session will help bring an effortless, single-minded focus as you dig deep into the psyche and the emotional wounding.

Surrounding a lapis with small blue sapphire crystals will amplify the third eye opening effects and intuitive awareness. Since this can be so strong, it is good to place a smoky quartz beneath the feet for balance and psychic and emotional strength. Wearing a blue sapphire as earrings or on the third eye will work well to stimulate your intuitive powers so you can use them in your emotional healing session. It is recommended that you have between one and four small blue sapphires.

Additional Emotional Healing Crystals and Stones

You will be able to do all your emotional healing with the crystals and stones described in the basic crystal healing kit. However, like adding

The Ultimate Guide to Emotional Healing with Crystals & Stones

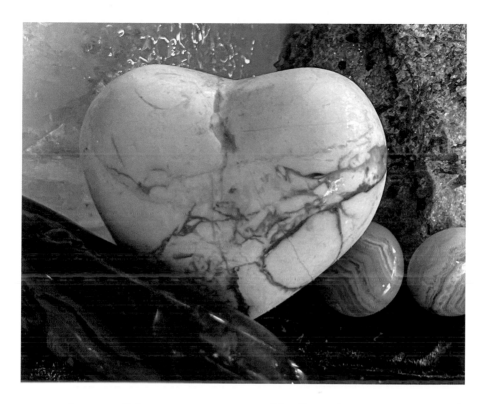

more spice to a dish, you may want to add a few other stones or crystals to "finetune" your kit, so that you can work with more nuance and further refine your work. Specifically, it is often helpful to refine your work by adding the extra uplift from the sky or the further nurturing of the earth. You may find that you need extra strength to open the heart if there is extra resistance. Or you may find that you need to help open the lungs to help the person in your emotional healing session breathe more freely since the breath and mental/emotional processes are intimately related to each other. You may find that you need to open the person to the higher awareness and expanded consciousness necessary to experience their unlimited self well beyond the emotional, mental, or physical. With emotions held within such an expanded perspective, joy then becomes their predominant experience, and their emotions no longer seem so overwhelming.

Here are some extra heart, earth, sky, and lung crystals and stones that you may want to add to your kit:

GREEN CRYSTALS AND STONES

The green crystals and stones are good to use when you want to help someone be more grounded into the earth, but not as deeply as they would be if you used your smoky quartz or black crystals and stones. Rather than deep into the earth, the green crystals and stones connect you more with nature, the plant life, flowers, grass, shrubs, and foliage of the earth. This connection with the vegetation of the planet connects you with their basic life force, their fecundity, and their quality. Connecting with the green plant world connects you with nurturing and mothering and is an excellent antidote to sadness.

Besides working with the healing of the physical heart, they will also work with the emotional aspect of the heart. The traditional color of the energetic heart energy center, green crystals and stones will also stimulate and open this center. Though rose quartz is the preferred color to work with the emotional aspects associated with the heart center, green can also be used, especially if someone suffers from early childhood wounding associated with a lack of mothering in any form. In this case, you may find it useful to lay a green crystal or stone on their heart center to help them feel mothered and accepted.

It is good to have at least four or five green crystals or stones in your emotional healing kit. That way you can place one on the heart center while you also surround the body with them. Here are some good ones that will work well:

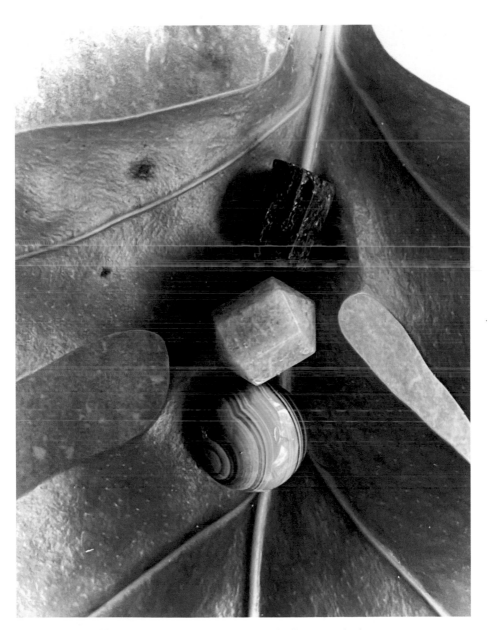

Natural Emerald Crystal, Green Aventurine, and African Malachite

GREEN AFRICAN MALACHITE

African malachite is a beautiful, bright, kelly green, usually with bands of darker green or black swirls. Because of its bright, dark, and pure green color, it is excellent to use when you feel the need for a major infusion of green energy, especially if you feel that you need the effects of green influence quickly. Perhaps, for example, the person you are working with is suddenly overcome with 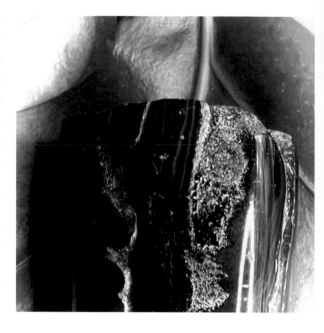 inconsolable grief from a core mother wound. In that case, you may want to place an African malachite on their heart center as you work to heal this wound. If you feel drawn to use this stone, you only need one for the heart center if you have other green crystals to surround the body when working with the nature elements.

GREEN CALCITE

Green calcite is a naturally occurring cubic crystal that is a light, soft, green color. It also works to help open the heart center. Where African malachite can be very intense in its effects, green calcite is quite gentle and envelops you with its soothing, kind, and restful energy. Because it is so calming and peaceful in its energy, it is also excellent to use when fiery and "hot" emotions like anger, anxiety, and fear need to be soothed and

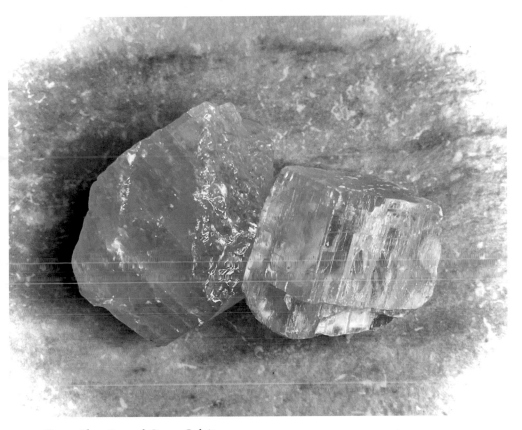

Green Fluorite and Green Calcite

rebalanced. For calming these emotions, you can place a green calcite on the heart center or on any place on the body in which these emotions are "stuck." If there is any place in the body that is retracted or tense as these and similar emotional states are expressed, place a green calcite on that area and have the person imagine breathing in the energy of the cool, soothing, green calcite and breathe out as they relax the tension. Green calcite is excellent to combine with rose quartz in your work with the heart center, as both are soothing and calming crystals.

It would be useful to have one good-sized green calcite in your crystal and stone emotional healing kit. An optimal size to use is approximately 1.5 by 1.5 inches. Then have four more that can be this size or smaller.

BLUE LACE AGATE

Blue lace agate is a quartz-based form of chalcedony that is light blue in color with white banding. Besides working with the physical healing of bones, the thyroid and throat, lymph system, and inflammation, blue

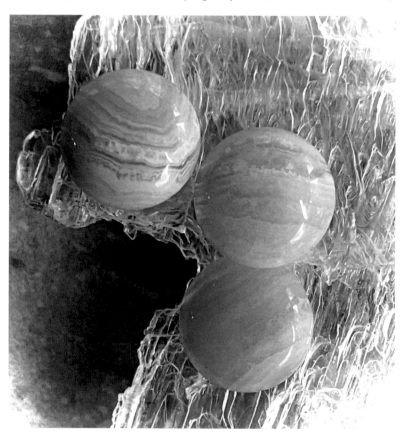

lace agate is known to uplift your overall sense of well-being. Associated with both air and water, it is a stone that feels tranquil, peaceful, and expansive. It will help bring these qualities to your emotional healing work. Immensely soothing, it is a great stone to work with any emotions that need calming. Because it also works with the throat energy center, it will help you or the person you are working with to put words to their emotions, helping to heal through their speaking. If difficult emotions are being repressed by incomplete or constricted breathing, or tightness in the chest or upper back, the application of blue lace agate to these areas will help relax them and free the emotions. Likewise, if someone that you are working with is babbling uncontrollably to keep you away, placing a blue lace agate on their throat center while you ask them to stop talking and breathe in and out of their throat center will help.

Though you can use other crystals to also help in these ways, a blue lace agate may be easier to use in some cases. You only need one or two pieces in your emotional healing kit. A tumbled stone rather than one that is raw or carved into a crystal shape is best because its roundness accentuates the stone's soothing quality.

WHITE HOWLITE

White howlite is a stone composed of hydrous calcium borate and is an opaque white with gray or black banding. Besides working bones, teeth, nails, and hair, white howlite is used to help balance calcium levels in the physical body. White howlite is used to bring stillness to your mind and increase your patience. It will help you sleep. It is also a calming stone for uncontrolled rage, anxiety, and other such turbulent emotional states. It is even more calming than green calcite and rose quartz. It is useful to use this stone in conjunction with the calcite and rose for tranquil heart energy. Besides being calming, it also helps stimulate or open the energy center of the crown. When you want to work to uplift depressive

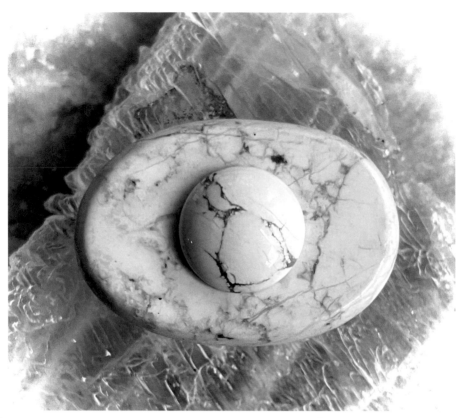

White Calcite on Selenite

emotional states or bring the ability to "see the larger picture," this is a good stone to use. Place it on the top of the head and imagine a white beam of expansive, inspiring, and calming angelic light flowing into the crown center to flood down through the entire body. As it does this, relax the entire body and imagine it filled with white light.

If you choose to have some white howlite in your emotional healing kit, choose two equal-sized pieces, either tumbled or in a cabochon form that is round with a flat bottom so that it can sit easily on the body. Place the stones on each lung point, on the chest above each nipple, or on the middle of the stomach to free constricted breathing caused by emotional stress and to release "stuck" fiery emotions. A good size to use for both cabochon stones is approximately 0.75 inches in diameter.

LEPIDOLITE

The lepidolite stone is from the group of mica minerals. Intermixed with these mica minerals, it contains concentrations of natural lithium. Ranging from pink to violet, or mixtures of these colors, it is thought to be the most relaxing stone used for emotional healing work because of its lithium content. Using this stone will cause immediate deep calming and relaxation. Because of the strength of this calming effect, it immediately calms unstable, chaotic, disordered, hostile, restless, or tumultuous emotional states. It can be placed on the heart center, the abdomen, or belly, held in the left hand, or placed prominently in the healing room or environment for immediate effects. However, it is not a good stone to lay on the body or have in your healing environment when you or the person you are working with is suffering from depression, grief, sadness, apathy, unhappiness, or confusion. Instead use green and pink crystals like rose quartz and green calcite.

If you feel drawn to include lepidolite in your crystal and stone emotional healing kit, either have a hand-sized natural or tumbled stone that is at least 2 inches in height by 1 inch wide. You can also use a lepidolite that is carved into a traditional six-sided crystal shape with a point on the end so you can use the stone to actively transmit this energy into the body. It is also useful to have a larger piece of lepidolite in your emotional healing room that is at least 4 inches square to create a calming, healing atmosphere. Remember, however, to remove it if you are working with any depressive states.

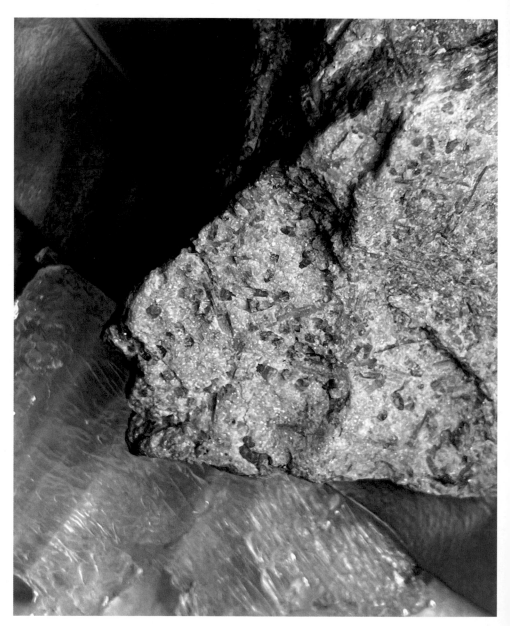

Lepidolite on Selenite

GARNET

There are many times in your emotional healing that you need to add fire energy to your work, especially when you are working with depressive states. When someone feels hopeless, overwhelmed, apathetic, withdrawn, sad, or other such state, you may need to balance them with the application of garnet. These depressive and other negative states feel cool and dull, gray-like in their energy, and can be countered with the vigor and intensity of fire energy.

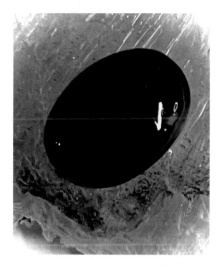

A red garnet is an excellent crystal to use for this. (You can use a ruby, red carnelian, red tourmaline, or red spinel if you don't have a garnet.) Related to the energy center at the base of the spine, garnet is said to channel basic life force into the physical, mental, and emotional bodies. This brings passion, vitality, warmth, and a sense of protection to the person wearing or holding the crystal.

For this reason, it is useful to include a red garnet in your emotional healing collection. If so, it should be a natural crystal at least 1 inch square or a cabochon stone that can be placed easily on the body. If you use a garnet cabochon, it should be round and at least 1 inch in diameter. An oval cabochon should be at least 1.25 inches in height and 0.5 inch in width. If you use a garnet that has been carved in the traditional six-sided shape, it should be at least 1.25 inches in height and 0.5 inch wide with a single termination so you can transmit energy in a direction that you determine.

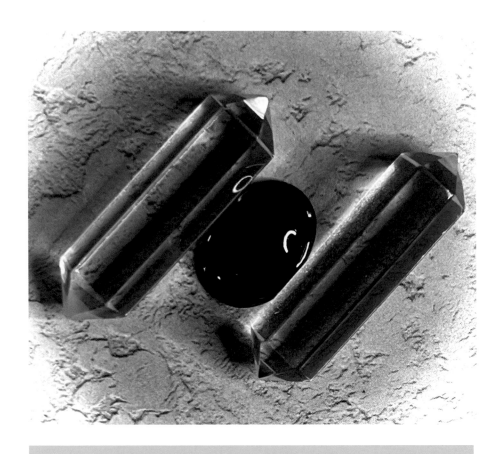

GARNET CRYSTAL TECHNIQUE TO BRING VITALITY

Here is a technique that you can use with your garnet that is quite powerful, as it brings these vital energies to the emotions:

1. Working with yourself or another person, hold a red stone to the body about 2 or 3 inches below the belly button or at the base of the spine.
2. Imagine a stream of red light flowing up the spine to fill the body with red light.

The Ultimate Guide to Emotional Healing with Crystals & Stones

3. As you do this, breathe with full, complete, breaths, filling and emptying the lungs. Each in-and-out breath should last between a half and full second. Don't breathe more rapidly to avoid hyper-ventilation.
4. If you feel light-headed at any time, relax and breathe regularly until you can resume.
5. Do this for three to ten minutes at the most since it is very powerful.
6. You can amplify the effects of this technique by holding a clear quartz crystal in each hand with its tip pointing up toward the arm.
7. Rest and let this fire light energy absorb into you and do its work. When you are through, be sure to clear your garnet crystal.

AMBER

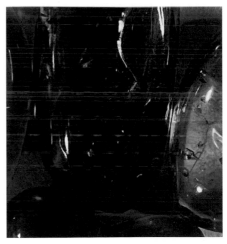

Amber, a form of fossilized tree sap formed eons ago, is very good to use when you need to add some fire energy but red garnet, or other red crystals, is too intense. Amber, containing mothering energy, can achieve the same effect but in a much gentler manner. Used for the physical healing of any female reproductive and other issues, amber will help bring a feeling of being protected, warmly nurtured, and totally accepted. Known to help foster the ability to manifest, it is helpful to use when feeling impotent, helpless, ineffective, or feeble in any way. Instead of despair, it will help bring a sense of hope and possibility.

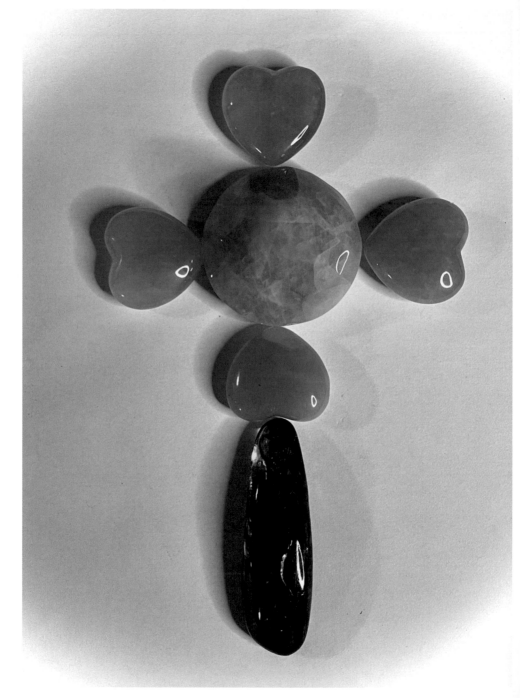

Crystal Layout to Balance the Heart with Personal Potency

You may want to add a piece of amber to your emotional healing kit to use when the garnet is too strong for the emotional system to handle.

BALANCING THE HEART WITH PERSONAL POTENCY

1. Lying on your back with your spine straight and your hands down by your sides, place an amber on your belly.
2. Place a rose quartz surrounded by four green crystals on your heart center.
3. Using long, deep breaths in and out of your nose, imagine the breath flowing in through the pink and green crystals and your heart center and out through the amber and your belly.
4. Then imagine the next breath flowing in through the amber and your belly and out through your heart center.
5. Do this for at least seven minutes. This will balance the emotions of your heart with a feeling of capability and personal potency.
6. When you are through, rest for another three minutes while experiencing this balanced energy.
7. Remove and clear your crystals after you arise.

If you want to add a piece of amber to your collection, it is best to use a tumbled or smooth piece that is at least 2 inches in height and 0.75 inches in width. The tumbled piece's smoothness will feel comforting, soothing, and reassuring.

OTHER VIOLET CRYSTALS

Amethyst is the best violet crystal to use in your emotional healing work because of its overall healing energy. However, you may want to augment the healing energy of this stone with some other violet crystals. When using another violet crystal, combine it with the amethyst by sitting it next to or on top of the amethyst. It is especially powerful

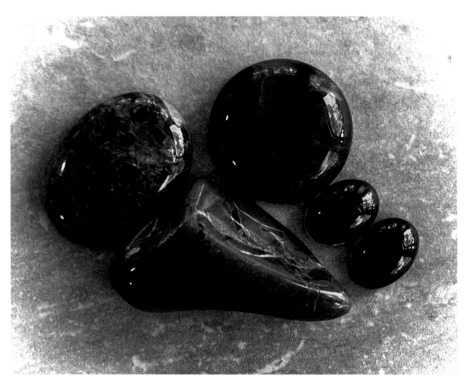

Charoite, Purple Fluorite, Iolite, and Sugilite

to place an amethyst over the crown energy center on the top of your head, then place the other violet crystal or crystals over the top of the amethyst so they are lined up straight above the head. This will greatly amplify the insight and higher awareness with which you can guide your healing.

Other violet crystals you may want to consider are violet charoite, purple sugilite, purple iolite, and purple fluorite. You must have amethyst in your emotional healing kit even though you may have one or more of these other crystals. They are used strictly to augment the effects of the amethyst. If you do use any one of these other purple crystals or stones, meditate with them first to learn what help they are specifically offering to you. You can keep them near you as you do your emotional healing session, and if you "hear" any of these crystals calling to you, or if you feel pulled by any one of these during your session, go ahead and use it. For your guidance, here is the list of other violet stones and what they are purported to do. Again, amethyst will do all the work that these crystals and stones can do, so they are strictly for you to use to augment the work you do with your amethyst.

Violet charoite is believed to bring divine inspiration, increase your sense of empathy, and bring the love of the Divine into your life. It is a good crystal to place on your heart chakra. You only need one of these in a small size.

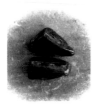

Purple sugilite is believed to generate positive energies and is known to help overcome negative emotions. Known as a strong psychic stone, it also helps bring peace of mind and relieve stress. It is also believed to offer release from the emotional trauma associated with past lives and bring emotional purification. Sugilite can be placed above the head on the crown energy center, placed on the heart center, or on the third eye. Choose one of these stones.

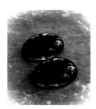

Purple Iolite is believed to be able to help you find your way when you are lost. If someone feels lost and overwhelmed in their life, it may be useful to place a purple iolite on their third eye chakra. It also is believed to help you widen your vision so that if you feel stuck in life, this may be a good stone to use. Choose one of these.

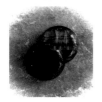 **Purple Fluorite** is another crystal that is known for its gentleness. It is thought to bring creative energy and help with lucid dreamwork as well as opening the crown energy center for divine inspiration and expanded consciousness. It can be placed anywhere on the body where trauma is stored so that it releases, as well as on the top of the head. You can surround your body with four of these for total relaxation.

SECTION FIVE
BEGINNING YOUR EMOTIONAL HEALING SESSION

The following techniques can be used for any type of emotional healing, no matter what the issue. Since you obviously don't use them all at the same time, the skill is in knowing which technique to use and when to use it. Each one of these techniques will be described with an example and picture so you will learn how to do them accurately. In that way, they will do their work. Each time that you use one of these techniques, your skill will improve as well as your sensitivity as to when to use it.

Beginning Your Emotional Healing Sessions

How you begin your emotional healing sessions with your crystals and stones is very important because it sets the mental/emotional tone for the following sessions and lets the other person know what to expect. It will also give you some information about the ease at which you will be able to work with someone and a beginning idea of the issues that you will be working with. Very importantly, it also attunes you to each other and starts building trust, both of which are essential to the success of your eventual healing.

BUILDLING TRUST WITHIN THE EMOTIONAL HEALING SESSION

No emotional healing work can be successful unless you are completely trusted by the person you are working with. Some people will trust you

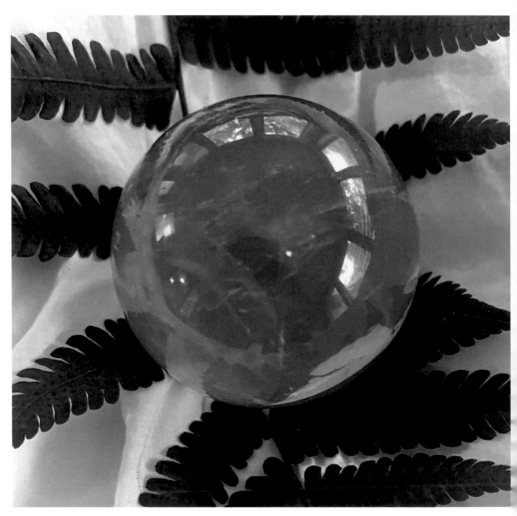

Rose Quartz Sphere

easily, while others will take a long time to open up enough to trust you. This largely depends on their basic personality as well as their past experiences. If they have been betrayed in the past, it will be harder for them to trust in the present.

The first work that you need to do in your emotional healing sessions is to create a sense of trust within the session. If your healing environment radiates a sense of peace, this is a good start. On the first session, you can surround the room or healing space with rose quartz, amethyst, green calcite or serpentine jade, live plants (make sure they're healthy), and comfortable chairs to sit on. If they are to be lying on the floor, make sure the cushion that they are on is comfortable, yet not so comfortable that they will fall right to sleep.

It is important to also let the person know how you will be working together during the sessions and some idea of the various techniques you will use together. This way, they will know what to expect and can comfortably relax.

Here are some basic instructions that will help you create a sense of safety and trust in your emotional healing sessions with your crystals and stones:

1. **Trust yourself.** If you don't trust yourself, neither will the other person. You need to trust that you will do the best you can for the other person. You need to trust that you will be honest with yourself, not try to be someone you are not. In fact, it is best not to try to be anyone at all. Just be yourself. You are fine as you are as long as you are sincere. Learn the various techniques given to you in this book, but at the same time, the most important thing you can do is learn to listen to your inner higher self, that river of knowledge and information that endlessly flows within you that is entirely accessible when you know how to listen. If your

higher energy centers are open, your heart is open, and if you are humbly willing, you will hear.

2. Part of creating a sense of safety in the healing environment is to feel safe yourself. If you don't feel safe with the other person before you begin working with them, don't work with them. If you aren't comfortable working with any of the behaviors or emotions that they present, then you are not the one to work with them. An example of this is violence. Some people are going to react with violence, rage, and other difficult emotions. Be sure that you know how to work with this.

3. Basically, any emotions you are not comfortable with within yourself, you will be unable to work with it in another. Therefore, it is important to do your own emotional healing work, not just once, but as long as you are offering emotional healing sessions. Emotional healing work is never done. Even if you are feeling peaceful and emotionally whole, there is always something deeper within to explore. We have no limits. There is always more to explore.

4. Always be truthful during the sessions and let the other person know that you are going to be truthful. Be truthful with discretion, however. Use words that you know they will be able to take in. Frame the truth as you experience it in a way that can be absorbed by the other. Use your words as a bridge rather than a bludgeon. Also, don't reveal a truth as you see it before the other is ready to hear. You will only create resistance and distrust.

5. Always be reliable. Part of that is having firm parameters that they can rely on. Start and end the session on time, every time. Refuse to accept emotional abuse from the other person. Model acceptable behavior. Firm parameters are the supports that will allow the other person to completely relax. They also model what works in interactions with others. Boundaries create comfort and

foster growth. The more they can rely on you, the more they can trust you.

6. Be transparent. Let the other person know how you feel and what you are experiencing during the session. That doesn't mean that you should start telling them about your life or your needs. Not only is that over-sharing, but it is counterproductive. By showing your feelings, you are modeling transparency and relationship. Don't hide from the other person. They will sense it. If you have a thought that needs sharing, share it. However, take responsibility, refusing to infer that it is the other making you think a certain way. A more appropriate response, instead, is something along these lines: "When you say that, I feel like this." Take responsibility for your own feelings. This models appropriate emotional sharing and will help them in their relationships. Timing is everything, however. Don't overwhelm the other by revealing too much too soon.

7. Truth builds trust. Always be truthful. Don't tell lies in any shape or form, even if it seems like it may be helpful. If you don't know something, it is okay to let them know that you don't know. Perhaps you can explore together.

8. Emotional healing that is done in the healing session is a mutual exploration, a journey that you are doing together. The more enthusiasm that you have, the more enthusiasm they will have. Ask them to join you in this exciting journey.

9. Show compassion without pity, no matter how bad you feel about what the other is going through. Pity is off-putting. Compassion is not. Pity puts you in a superior position while compassion holds you in mutual understanding.

10. Above all, be kind. Be kind in your communications. Be kind in your treatment of them. Let your understanding spring from your

open heart. Keep your heart open during the sessions. Kindness is healing just by itself.

There is no one stone or crystal to use to build trust, rather it is the way you conduct yourself during the session and how much trust you have in yourself and in your work. Building trust in your session is about your ability to open your heart and connect with the other person emotionally so that they feel completely safe with you and respected by you. Never create a one-up relationship with the person you are working with. Rather, hold and convey the attitude that you are engaged in a mutual exploration with them. Let them know that you are not the one with all the answers. Instead, you know the techniques through which they can find their own answers. Your focus should not be on yourself other than to reference what you experience and "see" during the session. Your focus, instead, is entirely on them. This is their process that you are here to assist them with. Let them know that they are unique and important to you.

You build a sense of trust through the sense of safety you create in your healing environment and the openness and genuine interest through which you approach and interact with the other person. You build trust when you let the other know that everything that they say in the emotional healing is completely confidential, that you will never betray, belittle, or disparage them in any way, neither in nor out of the emotional healing session.

AS THE OTHER PERSON IS HEALED, SO ARE YOU.

The Ultimate Guide to Emotional Healing with Crystals & Stones

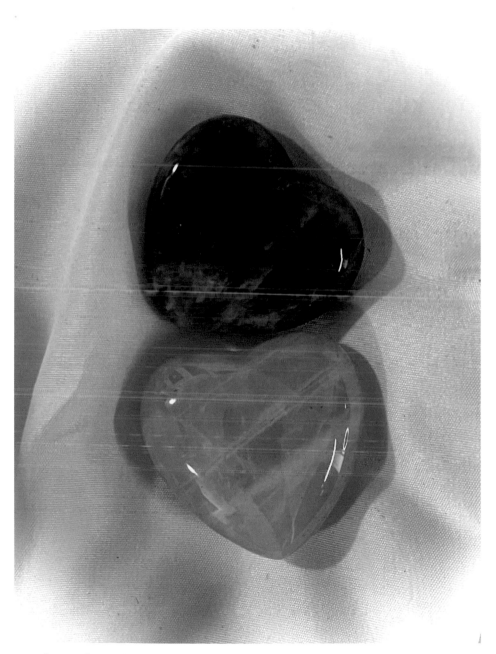

Amethyst and Rose Quartz

Basic Relaxation Technique with Crystals and Stones

One of the first techniques that you can do with the other person before you begin doing a series of emotional healing sessions is a relaxation technique. This will introduce the person to the use of crystals and stones and introduce yourself as the crystal emotional healer. This way they can get a feeling for what it would be like working with you, and you can start building a feeling of rapport and trust. You will also be able to get a feeling of what it will be like to work with that person. As you start doing this relaxation process with the other person, you may also start to receive some impressions about their emotional issues that you will be working with.

It is best to do a relaxation technique before you do any deep emotional work. This is one that you can use to prepare yourself before you begin any of your own emotional healing work. Often, when you find that you are in emotional turmoil, all you need to do is this relaxation technique to gain the insight that you need to calm and correct the upset.

Since the heart is your emotional center, this relaxation process begins and ends in your heart center. During your energy healing sessions, it is good to start the session by using a shortened version of this so that the other person's heart is open for good emotional access. Then you can end with a heart-opening relaxation process, as well, so they leave feeling happier than they started. As you place the various crystals and stones on and around the body, tell the person what you are doing and about the energy associated with the stone. For example, when you are laying a rose quartz on the heart center, say something like, "I am now laying a gentle, pink rose quartz on your heart center. This crystal will help open your heart to love and self-acceptance."

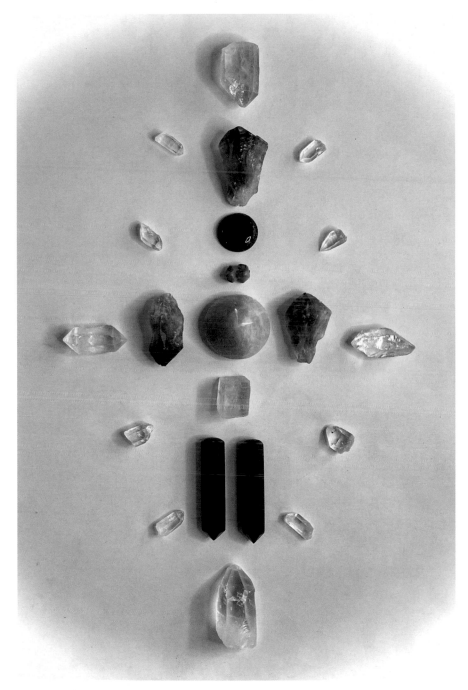

Crystal Layout for Relaxation

OPENING RELAXATION TECHNIQUE WITH CRYSTALS AND STONES

1. Have the person lie down on their back with their legs and arms uncrossed and their hands down at their sides with the palms upward. Ask them to close their eyes and let them know you will be laying crystals and stones on them and will let them know exactly what you are doing as you do it.

2. Start by placing a rose quartz on their heart energy center in the middle of their chest between the two breasts. As you place the rose quartz, have them breathe with long, slow, gentle, complete breaths and imagine that each in-breath flows into the heart center. Ask them to relax their body with every out-breath.

3. Place one or two smoky quartz crystals beneath the feet, asking the person to imagine or feel as if they are growing deep, gentle roots into the earth with every out-breath. As the roots grow deeper into the earth, ask them to relax the small of their back, their pelvis, the top of their legs front and back, then behind their knees, then their calves and shins. Again, with every out-breath, ask them to relax their feet and toes.

4. Now, place an amethyst over the top of their head, asking them to imagine that the top of their head opens and a gentle, amethyst beam of light flows up from their head into the heavens with every out-breath. As they do so, ask them to relax their forehead and their entire head.

5. Now, place a gentle yellow calcite or other yellow crystal about 2 inches below their belly button. As you do this, ask them to relax their stomach and the small of their back with every out-breath and imagine a gentle, warm, relaxing, joyful light flowing into the crystal and belly with every in-breath.

6. Place a small lapis or royal blue crystal or stone in the center of their forehead and ask them to relax their eyes, forehead (again), ears, and jaw with every out-breath. Ask them to let go or release any thoughts that they may be having and just rest.

(Continued on next page)

7. Now, place a small turquoise stone in the middle of their throat, asking them to imagine that a beautiful turquoise light flows into their throat with every in-breath and to relax their throat, jaw, upper chest, and upper back with every out-breath.

8. Next place an amethyst in each upward turned hand. If they are single terminated, point the tip upward toward the arm in the left hand. Point the tip outward in their right hand. After guiding them to relax their arms, hands, and fingertips with every out-breath, ask them to imagine that, with every in-breath, a gentle, healing, violet light flows into every part of their body and mind, and as it does, to relax even more with every out-breath.

9. Surround their body with clear quartz crystals with their tips pointing outward from the body. Place them about a foot apart from the body's surface. You can use four; one pointing upward from the head, one below the feet, and one at each side of the body.

10. Ask them to shift their focus to their heart center while maintaining their state of relaxation and imagine that they are surrounded in a halo of clear, angelic light.

11. As they do this, ask them to breathe in and out of their heart center. If they get distracted from their focus on their heart center, ask them to let any thoughts go and bring their attention to the heart center. If you notice any area of tension remaining in their body, ask them to relax that.

12. Stay in this state of relaxation for at least ten minutes. When you are through, while asking them to continue relaxing with every out-breath, slowly remove each crystal in the reverse order in which you placed them on and around the body. Remove the heart crystal last.

13. When you are through, ask them to rise and see if they can maintain the same state of awareness and relaxation as they had during this process.

After this process, you can both be seated. Ask them if any thoughts or feelings arose for them during this process. If so, have them describe them; what they were, and where they were felt in the body. If they cannot feel them in their body, ask them to imagine where they might be felt in their body. Ask if these feelings are familiar to them, if they are reoccurring, and if they would be willing to concentrate on these later in this session or in following sessions. Besides being relaxing, this will help them open to their emotional experience and provide a starting point with which to start their emotional healing sessions.

During this process, you will find yourself becoming mentally quieter, more centered, more attuned to yourself and the other person. Then you will be able to intuit some of the emotional issues that they are dealing with.

Once you start each one of your emotional healing sessions, start with at least an abbreviated relaxation technique so that not only are they relaxed, which allows for more emotional attunement, but also so you attune with each other and that both of you are completely centered in the present. Then start your session with this question: "How are you feeling right now?"

ALL HEALING HAPPENS WHEN COMPELTELY CENTERED IN THE PRESENT.

Ways to Use Your Crystals and Stones for Emotional Healing

These are the main ways that you can use your crystals during an emotional healing session:

1. Laying the stones or crystals on the body
2. Creating crystal energy grids and healing patterns

3. Creating an emotional healing energy field or aura teamed with visualization and crystal and stone empowerment

Here is how each one of these is accomplished:

HOW TO LAY CRYSTALS AND STONES ON THE BODY

This is one of the main ways that the crystals and stones are used during a healing session. This method uses the vibration of the stones to interact with and change the vibrational pattern of the one being healed from one supporting emotional pain to one supporting emotional healing. You can remove the pain of emotional trauma by creating a new vibrational pattern within the body and mind that matches one of harmony. When you do this, negative emotions tend to positively transform. If someone is feeling angry, for example, the energetic vibrations of their body and mind may feel rapid, jagged, intense, and appear red to the mind's eye. To change the anger to peace, you can use your crystals and stones to change the vibrational pattern to one that matches calmness, perhaps slowing the rate of vibration and shifting the red that is seen in the mind's eye to green. As you do this, the angry feelings should calm.

Sometimes you can do this in one session if the emotion is not deep-seated but one based on a particular event. Quite often, however, it is a response that is more rooted in past events and the subconscious decisions about life and themselves that they have made in the past. These, in turn, affect them in the present. If that is the case, you not only work to change the vibrational pattern, but in doing so, you discover the source of the emotional pain and work to change those dynamics. as well. You may find yourself changing the crystals you place on the body as you reveal these deeper levels one by one and shift their vibrational patterns accordingly. In that way, shifting vibrational pattern is not a one-shot process, but one that may take many sessions as each emotional layer is revealed.

For example, perhaps someone comes to you who wants to stop feeling so sad. In your mind's eye, you see this sadness as a dull-gray vibrational pattern that is quite sluggish. Your first thought may be to lay some yellow crystals on the body that match a more joyful expression. However, then you may discover that underlying the sadness is a subconscious decision and resulting feeling that people can never be trusted. Then, as that is revealed, you work with shifting the vibrational pattern to one that supports trust, perhaps working with earth-colored grounding, rose quartz, and violet crystals. But what then may be revealed underlying the mistrust is fear, so then you may want to lay crystals on the body that shift the fear state to strength. Finally, when you, or the person you are working with, feels strong and less fearful, you can remove those crystals and just use your yellow crystals that help create the joyful feeling that they are now able to accept and relax into. This will be further explained as you read about specific emotional healings later in this book.

When you lay a crystal or stone on the body, you don't just plop it down. Instead, the crystal must be accepted by the person being healed. It isn't that they say something like, "I accept this crystal," although sometimes someone will have such an aversion to one stone or another being laid on their body that they will physically shy away from it or actually tell you that they don't like it. Normally, when you lay a stone or crystal on the body, you approach it carefully. Here is how you do it:

First, make sure that you won't be interrupted and that the environment feels safe for the person you are working with. Next, center and ground yourself. Then shift your attention to your sense of inner knowing beyond your rational mind and individual ego, a state explained in the beginning of this book. Help the person you are working with relax and center themselves with some long, deep breathing in and out of their heart center. Have them close their eyes as they do this and let themselves open into a state of acceptance. You may ask them if they are willing to accept the crystals and stones that you will lay on their body. If so, then you sensitize your hands. If you like, you can hold a clear quartz crystal or a Herkimer diamond in your left hand as a receptive crystal so that it helps you receive information as you do the work. If this crystal is single terminated, point the tip up toward your arm.

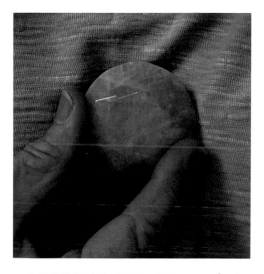

Now that you and the other person are prepared, start by placing a rose quartz on their heart center. Holding the first rose quartz crystal or stone in your right hand, slowly approach the body with the it. Let the person you are working with know which crystal you are using. As you reach the area upon which you intend to lay this first crystal, first hold it about 4 to 6 inches above the body in that heart area, never letting your attention wander. As you focus, you will feel a buoyancy, or a feeling that somewhat resembles "thick air." Contact that, and then slowly begin to lower the crystal through the buoyancy. If it is accepted, it will easily go through onto the skin of the body. Then place the next crystal on the body where you feel that it should go. Anytime that the crystal or stone is not the right one to be used, or it isn't the right time to use it, you will have a very slight feeling of the stone or crystal being repelled or almost bouncing back. In that case, don't force the crystal or stone down onto the body because either it isn't the right crystal or stone to use, or it is the wrong time to use it. Ask the person you are working with how they are feeling at that moment, perhaps letting them know that that crystal or stone doesn't seem to want to be used. Ask the person how they are feeling as that happens. Don't ask them *why* because you don't want them to start trying to "figure out"

Beginning Your Emotional Healing Session

anything or otherwise get caught up in their thinking mind. You may ask them how they *feel* about that. They may or may not have feedback. Next, see if you intuit another stone or crystal that should be used. Or wait for a few moments and try the same crystal or stone again and see if it's accepted. Once you have laid the first stone on the body, let it sit for a few moments and then repeat this same process to lay another crystal or stone on the body. Keep doing this until you have all the crystals or stones laid on the body.

Laying a stone on the body and working with its acceptance or resistance doesn't have to take a long time. In fact, usually the acceptance of a stone or crystal happens rather quickly. There is a flowing, graceful quality to this process. You may find yourself moving around the other's body with incredible grace, almost as if you are doing a dance. You may find that you sing, hum, or make sounds. You may also find that your eyes automatically roll upward and start focusing on your third eye in the middle of your forehead between your brows. If these things happen, go ahead and let them. Don't resist or you will stop the flow.

If you pay attention, you will feel their vibrational energy shift as the crystals do their work. As they do their work, let the person simply rest with the stones and crystals on them. In fact, sometimes they fall asleep. It is okay if they do this, because the stones and crystals are still doing their work. After all, the crystals are still vibrating in their usual patterns whether or not the person is asleep. At least when the person is asleep, they are in a receptive rather than a resistant state so the healing may actually happen more quickly.

If you are attuned, you will get a definite feeling when it is time for the crystals and stones to be removed from the body. If you don't receive an intuitive feeling that it is time to remove the stones and crystals, let them remain on the body for at least twenty minutes or even longer if it seems that they need to be. Once you are done, you generally remove the crystals and stones in the reverse order in which

The Ultimate Guide to Emotional Healing with Crystals & Stones

you placed them. This isn't a hard and fast rule, however. If you are attuned, you may find that the crystals and stones seem to want to be removed in a different order. If so, pay attention to that and then remove them in this order. Before you remove the crystals and stones, let the person know that you are going to do this. (Gently wake them if you must do so.) Then let them know which crystals you are moving. Take your time; there is usually no hurry. As you remove the various crystals and stones, lift each one up gently, again feeling the buoyancy between them. When you do, remove the crystal by gently raising it upward while remaining in contact with the buoyancy until you don't feel it anymore. (It feels as if the crystal or stone releases itself.) Always leave a crystal, usually rose quartz, on the heart center to be removed last so that the process ends with the person's heart chakra open. When you have all the crystals removed, use a clear quartz in your right hand to sweep down the body, about 6 inches from its surface, to seal the healing. Sweep from left to right over the heart center so that it is not so wide open that the person isn't wide open or inappropriately takes on someone's energy.

It is important to remember when you do this healing work, that the other person you are working with is an important part of the process. While you are laying the crystals on their body, ask them if they are having any mental images or feelings come to them. If so, ask them to describe what they are "seeing" or feeling. As they relay these thoughts or images to you, you may find that you want to lay more crystals and stones on their body or shift the ones that are on there to different places on their body or remove them altogether. As you do this, continue to communicate to them what you are doing and why. It is important to realize that when you are laying stones or crystals on someone's body, it isn't something that you are doing *to* them, but instead it is something that you are doing *with* them. It is a mutual communication.

CRYSTAL HEALING IS DONE *WITH* THE PERSON RATHER THAN *TO* THEM.

As you lay the various stones and crystals on the other's body, you may have images appear in your mind's eye, receive intuitive messages about their emotional state, receive realizations about what may underlie their emotional pain, and so on. As you do so, relay these realizations to the person you are working with. You may just relay these helpful messages to them, or you may ask them if this resonates with them or makes sense to them. If you are working from the vantage point of oneness or higher consciousness, you will know when to speak, and if and when to have a dialogue with them. Or you may intuit that it is better to be silent so that your and their concentration isn't broken. Or you may even decide that it is better to let them sleep so that they remain receptive. You can always relay to the other person what it is that you "saw" or realized and have a discussion later when you both can process the information. In short, laying crystals and stones on the body is not a passive process but a mutual exploration to the heart of their emotional world.

Finally, it is important to realize that as you do this form of vibrational healing with your crystals and stones, you are in an altered state of expanded awareness. (If you are doing it correctly.) Instead of referring to your rational mind, you are paying attention to other ways of knowing that are far beyond the intellect. The more you do this work, the more easily you will be able to move beyond the rational into more expanded states of awareness. Immersed in this state, you receive information that flows through your being like an endless river of knowing. It is as if you lose your sense of separation from the other entirely so that there is just one being.

The Ultimate Guide to Emotional Healing with Crystals & Stones

> ## WE ARE ONE.
> ## SEPARATION BETWEEN US IS ILLUSORY.

CRYSTAL HEALING PATTERNS

The patterns in which we set the crystals and stones when emotional healing are generally those that follow the subtle energy pathways in the subtle body. They may be laid in a straight line vertically up the body or centered around one or more of the subtle energy pathways or center.

There is a central cord of energy, roughly in alignment with your spinal cord, that runs from the area near your tail bone, up your body, and out the top of your head. In this central cord of subtle life force energy are seven main chakras or centers of subtle energy, each regulating the areas of the physical and subtle body in its area. This central cord of energy also flows down into the earth from beneath your tailbone and bottoms of your feet. It also extends upward from the crown to flow into the heavenly realms.

> ## WE ARE NEITHER SEPARATE FROM THE EARTH NOR THE HEAVENS.
> ## ALL IS ONE.

For physical and emotional health, we need to have all these subtle energy centers activated and in balance with each other. You will often find that the emotional healings offered here in this book follow stimulating one or more of these energy centers. For example, since fear and anxiety affect your stomach and weaken your nervous system, you will find that crystal layouts that help this emotional issue tend to rest on or near your navel center that regulates the physical and subtle nervous

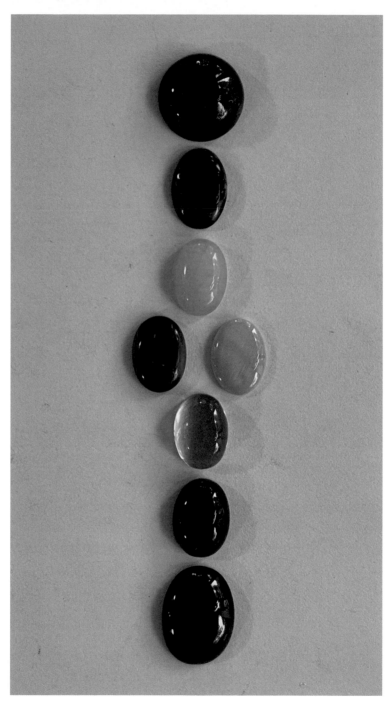

Basic Chakra Opening and Balancing Crystal Layout

system and works on the stomach. Similarly, grief either overstimulates or under-stimulates your heart center, so crystals or stones are often laid over the heart.

The following is a brief explanation of these subtle energy centers (called chakras) and the emotions that they predominantly work with. For a more detailed explanation of the chakra system, refer to my book *The Ultimate Guide to Crystals & Stones*.

The **first chakra** or energy center, its color red, works with basic survival, grounding, vitality, and feelings of safety.

The **second chakra** or energy center, its color orange, works with sexuality and sensuality, manifestation, intimacy, connections with others, passion, and enjoyment.

The **third chakra** near the belly button, its color yellow, works with issues of power, the nervous system, self-esteem, willpower, sense of purpose, and personal identity.

The **fourth chakra**, the heart chakra, is in the middle of your chest, roughly between your nipples. Its traditional color is green, although pink, the color of love, is most used with this center in emotional healing work. This subtle energy center is the one you almost always use in your emotional healing work, as it is associated with love, empathy, compassion, acceptance of self and others, forgiveness, and joy. Generally, when you are emotionally troubled, the heart chakra is deeply affected, usually overstimulated or closed to one degree or another.

The **fifth chakra**, its color turquoise blue, is centered in the middle of the throat. This center has to do with all forms of communication, self-expression, and the ability to find the words to speak your personal truth, hearing another, and being heard.

The **sixth chakra** is found in the middle of your forehead between your eyebrows. Its color royal blue, it is concerned with intuition, intellect, inner wisdom, and psychic vision, or connection with other ways of knowing beyond the intellect.

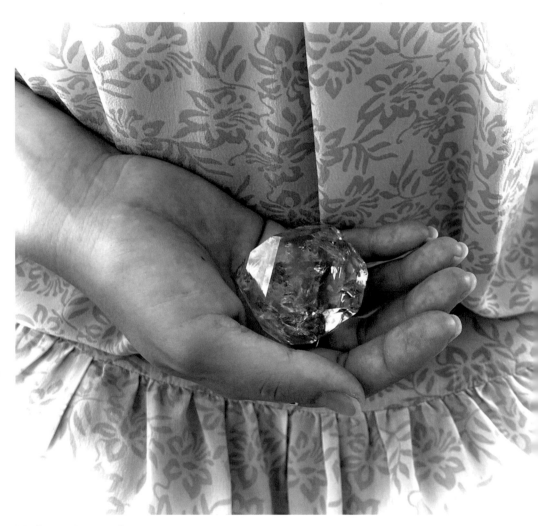

Herkimer Diamond

The **seventh crown chakra**, its color purple or pure white light, connects you with your higher self, the Higher Spirit, and brings divine vision and perspective. Its stimulation brings peace with a clear perspective. When it is blocked, you may experience disillusionment, boredom, despondency, sorrow, dejection, and restlessness. (There are other more minor energy centers in the subtle body. However, these are the main ones that you will work in your emotional healing.)

There are also energy centers, or chakras, in the middle of your palms that are important to know about. The more open these are, the more you will be able to feel the subtle energy of the crystals, in the body, and in the healing environment. If you are concentrated as you work with your crystals and stones, these will automatically open more and more. If you want to speed up this process, you can concentrate on your hands as you vigorously rub them together until you feel quite a bit of heat. Then, without dropping your concentration, pick up a bright, clear, quartz crystal and touch its tip lightly to your palm. Still concentrating, slowly pull the crystal up from your hand an inch or so. Then, circle the crystal clockwise in the middle of your palm. You should eventually feel a slight buzzing sensation, or a feeling of buoyancy between the crystal and your hand. If you don't feel this, do it again until you do. You may not feel it right away, but if you keep doing it, you eventually will.

Though these subtle energy centers tend to rule a certain set of emotions, you will find in your work that seldom is just one energy center affected. One or more of these energy centers are involved in varying degrees. When working with emotional transformation, it is not enough to just lay stones or crystals on the body. Almost always you will find that you also need to interact verbally with the other person with questions, observations, and guidance to find what other centers are affected. If you are working with yourself, you will also find that you need to question yourself. As you read about some of the emotional healings following this, you will see how this is done.

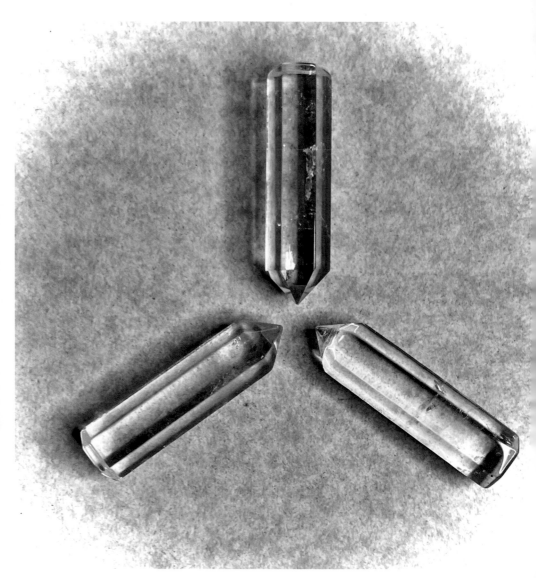

Clear Quartz Crystal Charging Pattern

Other patterns that are helpful to use in your emotional healing work are circles, squares, and triangles. Placing the crystals in a circle around the body will help provide a sense of protection, amplify the effects of what you are doing, and bring certain energies into the entire body rather than just one place. A square is often used to represent the four elements of earth, fire, water, and air. It can also represent the four seasons, winter, spring, summer, and fall, as well as the four domains of the spiritual, emotional, physical, and mental. It is thought that when the four sides of the square are all equally represented, we are balanced human beings. Placing a crystal or stone in each of these directions, or in the four corners of your healing space, can help bring all these elements to play in your emotional healing work. You can also place more crystals or stones in one direction or another if you want to bring more of its associated energy to bear in your work. If the person's emotions need cooling, for example, you may want to bring in more of the winter energy. Triangles are used when you want to add direction to your work. Generally, the energy tends to run from the bottom to the tip of the triangle. So, if you want to send energy, you place the triangle with its tip pointing outward from the body. Likewise, if you want to receive a particular energy, you point the triangle inward.

When you want to use your crystals in a square or triangle formation, you place each crystal or stone on each one of the corners and then imagine that they are each connected by a golden light. You can either imagine or visualize this alone, or you can amplify your visualization by using your clear crystal to trace this line of energy with its tip, holding it in your right hand. Usually, you trace this line of energy in a clockwise direction. If you want to undo this formation, you use your crystal in a counterclockwise direction as you visualize the line of energy disappearing. Then remove the crystals or stones in the reverse order in which you laid them down. If you are working with another person, you can either involve them in this visualization or not. It can be more powerful, however, to involve them.

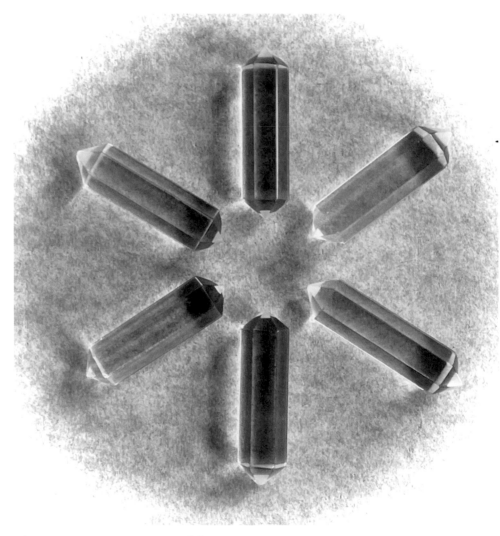

Clear Quartz Protection or Amplification Pattern

A good way to amplify the effects of your healing, or to bring a sense of protection to the person you are working with, is to surround their body in a circle of crystals or stones. You can do this if they are lying down, sitting, or standing. Generally, it is more balancing to use an even number of crystals or stones. As you place the crystals or stones in a circle, the technique is the same as placing them in the other formation. If the person is sitting or standing, start by placing a crystal in front of the body, then moving clockwise, place one on the right side of the body, behind it, and then on its left side. If you have more crystals, start at the front of the body, then put two on each side, or a crystal in between the initial four. If the person is laying down, start laying the circle of crystals over their head, then beneath their feet, and then fill in the circle with the rest of the crystals, moving clockwise as you lay the rest of the crystals. Generally, the smaller your crystals or stones, the more you will need to use to surround the body so that you have the degree of amplification that you want. Just as you did in the other formations, once you have laid down the stones or crystals, visualize a golden line of energy moving in a clockwise direction connecting each stone. When you are removing the circle, first visualize removing the connecting line of golden light in a counterclockwise direction and then remove the crystals in the reverse order in which you laid them down.

VISUALIZATION AND AFFIRMATION

Usually when you work with emotional healing, you not only lay stones and crystals on the body, but you combine it with visualization techniques and affirmations. Whether you are using visualization or affirmations, or a combination of both, they amplify the effects of the crystals or stones. The crystals and stones also amplify the effects of the visualizations and affirmations. Both visualizations and affirmations are designed to help the person you are working with discover the source of the emotional upset, to change their belief systems, subconscious decisions, and other dynamics that keep the upset in place. These are then replaced with alternative beliefs or decisions that change the reactive behaviors that maintain the negative emotion or emotional patterns. Then more pleasant or happier feelings are introduced in their place.

Visualizations, sometimes underrated, are actually very powerful tools to work with and can help make lasting change. It is easy to dismiss them as "just imagination." However, the mind is not unable to distinguish the difference between what is "real" or imagination. To the mind, it is all "real." The more powerful and concentrated the visualization, the more powerful it will be. Also, the more accurate you can pinpoint the core issue that keeps the upset in place, the more accurate visualization you can design to counteract it. If someone has debilitating shyness, for example, during your emotional healing work you may discover that it is tied to a feeling of underlying unworthiness. If so, your most powerful visualization may be one that helps the person feel worthy.

THE MIND DOESN'T DISTINGUISH BETWEEN THE REAL AND THE IMAGINARY. TO THE MIND IT IS ALL REAL.

Visualizations can be done to channel in color, light, and sound, introduce feelings, open energy centers, and imagine transformational actions. You don't have to use the word "visualization" during your healing. Sometimes it is more effective to use the word "imagine." Since you and the person you are working with are in an altered, concentrated state when you do the visualization, the rational brain is not available to think that anything is impossible. In that way, there is no limit to what can be visualized. When leading someone through a visualization, you must be careful to not be overly threatening or insensitive to their comfort level or you will find them leaving the visualization. That said, if you are introducing a new behavior or feeling that can be scary for them, then you must do it very carefully, backing off if you feel them pulling away from the visualization. If the person is afraid of large men, for example, you might surround the person with black tourmaline and have them imagine feeling very safe and powerful when they see a large man far in the distance. As the man gets closer and closer, they feel stronger and stronger, so much so that by the time the man gets close, he has shrunk down to be only knee high.

Affirmations are a way to retrain the way that the mind thinks so that negative thoughts are replaced by positive ones. These positive statements are ways for you to challenge and overcome thoughts and beliefs that are self-sabotaging or negative. The more you can transform these thoughts and beliefs, the more positive and capable you will feel. Like visualization, they are usually introduced while the person being healed is in an altered state so that they penetrate deeply. After introducing an affirmation, it works well to have the person being healed repeat the phrase or sentence after the healing session to reinforce the work that has been done. In the case of the person being afraid of large men, you might have them repeat, "I am powerful. I cannot be harmed."

IT IS ALL IMAGINED.

SECTION SIX
HEALING TECHNIQUES FOR COMMON EMOTIONAL UPSETS

The following painful emotions are the ones that you will find to be more prevalent in your work. Learning about the ways to treat the emotional upsets presented below will enable you to extrapolate and treat all the others with which you may be presented. These emotional states may be either deep-seated or more temporary states. Both of these will be addressed as each emotional state is presented here. The method being used with each of the emotional states is not the only method that you can use. They are, however, ones that work. As you try these, you will likely find variations that work for you. The methods presented below will include both the crystal or stone layouts as well as accompanying visualizations and affirmations.

Each of these healings begins with the same preparation: Begin with centering and grounding yourself. Sensitize your hands to the crystal energy. Shift your attention to your intuitive mind or expanded awareness. Breathing with long, deep breaths, take a few moments and feel as if you and the person you are working with are not separate but joined in oneness in the way that was illustrated in the opening chapters of this book. The more that you can do this, the more you will be in an alternate, expanded state of awareness beyond the rational mind. (You can do this without taking on their emotions.) Have the person you are working with preferably lay down on their back with arms and legs uncrossed and their palms upward in receptive position. Have them close their eyes and begin breathing with long, deep breaths in and out of their heart chakra in the middle of their chest until they feel centered.

Common Emotional Problems

ANGER

Anger is primarily manifested in the solar plexus, tight jaw, and generally depletes the nervous system, especially if it is deep-seated and has been happening a long time. It also closes the heart so that love, acceptance, and empathy is impossible to experience. It may also physically manifest itself as a tight chest or pain in the upper or mid back. It may also cause pain in the forehead, stomach, and throat. Since it is an emotion that feels hot, generally you want to provide coolness. Here is a suggested crystal and stone formation, visualization, and affirmation that you can use:

CRYSTAL AND STONE TECHNIQUE FOR ANGER RELIEF

1. Surround the body with rose quartz and hold a rose quartz in each hand. Place a green calcite or other green crystal on the heart energy center in the middle of the chest to both open the heart and provide coolness to the energetic body. Have them breathe in and out of their heart center, imagine a cool, green light entering their heart center as they relax their chest. Imagine that this cool, green light fills their entire body.
2. Place a light-yellow calcite or citrine on the belly button. This will help energize and repair the subtle nervous system. Have them relax their belly and small of their back as they do this, allowing the soft yellow light to fill their belly.
3. Place a smoky quartz beneath the feet with its tip pointing down into the earth. Have the person now imagine that their breath flows in through their heart center and down their body and out of their feet

(Continued on next page)

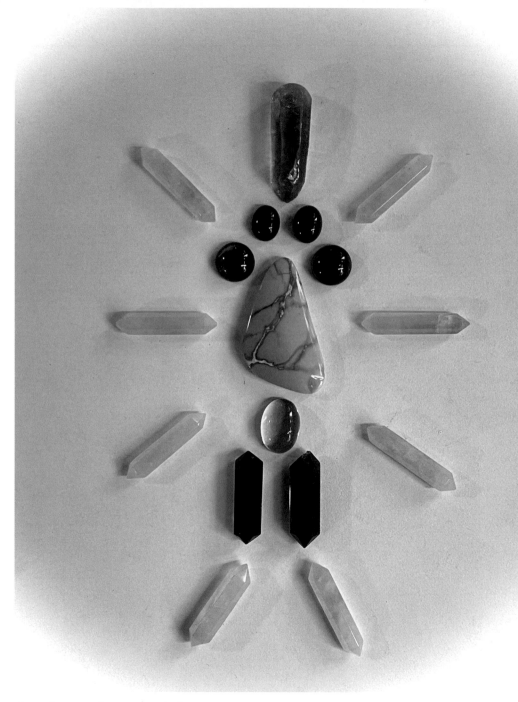

Crystal Layout for Anger Relief

with every exhale. Have them visualize long, deep, soft earth-colored roots flowing into the earth from the bottoms of their feet. With every exhale, these roots extend deeper and deeper into the earth.

4. Now, place a small amethyst over each temple as they shift their breathing back to their heart center. Have them continue to breathe with long, deep, gentle, and full breaths. As you place an amethyst on each temple, have them relax their forehead and jaw with every out-breath. If they are having trouble doing this, you may place another small amethyst on each side of their neck between their ears and shoulder.

5. Place an amethyst over the crown energy center at the top of the head. As you do this, have the person imagine that a violet stream of light flows down from the heavens to fill their head and then flow down through their entire body as they relax even further. Suggest that this will help bring a more expanded perspective to them.

6. Now guide the person to visualize themselves as being surrounded in a soft pink orb of light that also fills their entire body. At their center is a glowing, soft circle of cool, green, nurturing light of Mother Earth. Have them imagine that they breathe this soft, pink-green light into the heart of their being.

7. Now ask them to describe their anger without giving reasons why they are angry. Just let you know what the feeling of this anger is, where else they can imagine it in their body, and what color they can imagine it being. If they could see it, what would it look like? What color would it be? Do they see any images in their mind's eye as they imagine the color of this anger? As they tell you this, scoop this anger out from wherever they imagine it to be in their body and send it into Mother Earth. Scoop out any images as they are relayed to you. Let them know that you are doing this, suggesting that they feel lighter and lighter as you do it.

(Continued on next page)

8. Now ask them if they are willing to let this anger pass from them *at this time*. If so, ask them to imagine that they pass this anger into the middle of a ball of pink light. Once the anger is entirely held in this ball of light, have them imagine that it rises into the sky, getting further and further away until they cannot see it. Continue to suggest that they relax more and more, especially if you notice that their body is becoming tense at all. As they do this, use your clear quartz crystal in a scooping motion to help remove the anger and place it in the pink ball of light. Let them know that you are helping them by doing this.

9. If they are unwilling to let the anger go, ask them, *just this time,* to imagine the unwillingness as gray light that they place in the middle of a ball of clear light. Ask them to let the unwillingness go to float upward and upward until they cannot see it anymore. As you do this, use your clear quartz crystal to scoop the unwillingness from their heart center and place it in the clear ball of light. Describe what you are doing as you are doing it.

10. Next, ask them if they are willing to also let the anger go, just this time, and have them visualize it being placed in the pink ball of light that rises upward until it disappears. Again, scoop out the anger from their heart center with your clear crystal and put it in the pink ball of light. Describe to them what you are doing. Continue to have them relax.

11. Next, ask them if they could place another feeling in their heart center that would feel better. (Avoid mentioning their former anger.) Ask them to describe this feeling. Ask them how they feel having this feeling. Ask them to describe what color would it be if this feeling had a color. As they are telling you this, send this color into their heart center, letting them know that you are doing this. Have them breathe this color and feeling into their heart center with every breath, continuing to relax even further.

12. Ask them to just relax with this new feeling, breathing in and out of their heart center. As they do so, ask them to silently repeat, "I am peaceful. I am accepting." Relax and repeat this affirmation for at least seven minutes. They can do it longer than this if they choose.

13. Once you are through, remove the crystals in the reverse order in which you laid them on the body, letting the person know you are doing this. End with the crystal in the heart center, then remove that one.

14. Ask them to see if they can maintain this peaceful feeling and repeat the affirmation as they go about their day.

I AM PEACEFUL.
I AM ACCEPTING.

This process will help change the angry state to one of acceptance and peace. If the anger is a temporary feeling rather than one that results from deep-seated wounding, you may need to do it only once or twice, teaching them how to do it for themselves. If it results from deep-seated wounding, you will have to do this possibly combined with other stone layouts for every layer of wounding you uncover.

ANXIETY

Anxiety is basically related to fear. Rather than fear from something that is happening in *the present,* it results from what you imagine may happen *in the future.* Anxiety, then, cannot happen if your attention is centered in the present. The work with anxiety is to help the person center their attention to the present moment.

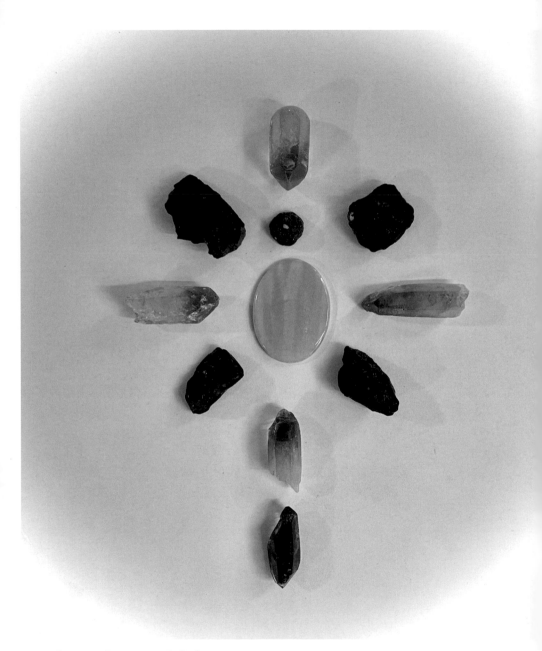

Crystal Layout for Anxiety Relief

When you feel anxious, your breathing becomes shallow and rapid, your body tenses, your heart rate increases. You may feel tired or even completely exhausted. You may have difficulty concentrating and feel constantly on edge. Your jaw, shoulders, and neck tighten, and you may feel pain on your back between your shoulder blades.

You may feel anxious when you are in certain situations, like public speaking or taking a test, but this anxiety is temporary and goes away when you are no longer in that situation. Anxiety, however, becomes a problem when these feelings become all-consuming, excessive, and interfere with your daily living. This is the type of anxiety that needs healing.

Physical activity will help combat anxiety, as well as a healthy diet, regular sleep, and the avoidance of caffeine, alcohol, and nicotine. It will also help to practice centering with long, deep breathing and to learn to replace reoccurring anxious thought patterns with positive ones. Some anxiety conditions are so severe and debilitating that you will also need to team your efforts with a medical professional. If this is the case, the work that you do with your crystals and stones can augment their work.

This crystal and stone healing that helps you become desensitized to the anxiety-producing event or events and become present-centered will also help:

CRYSTAL MEDITATION FOR ANXIETY RELIEF

1. Have the person you are working with lay on their back. Center and ground yourself, shifting your attention to your higher consciousness beyond your rational mind.
2. Surround the person with alternating black tourmalines or other black crystals and amethysts. These are for bringing a sense of protection, bringing a sense of capability, and relaxation. Use eight crystals, placing the amethyst over the head, an amethyst at each

(Continued on next page)

side, and one below the feet. Place the black crystals in between the amethysts. If they are terminated, point their tips in toward their body. Have the person hold an amethyst in each hand, if terminated, its tip pointing up toward their arm. Place a rose quartz or other pink crystal on their heart center for self-acceptance. Now place a smoky quartz beneath the feet just beyond the amethyst for grounding. Place a small blue azurite on the third eye center in the middle of the forehead for insight. The person can watch you do this as they listen to what you say about each crystal. Once you have laid all the crystals and stones around and on their body, have them close their eyes.

3. Have the person being healed breathe in and out of their heart center with gentle, deep breaths until they feel calm and even more centered. Have them imagine the pink of the rose quartz entering their body and filling it with peace with every breath.

4. Now have them imagine the amethyst crystals that surround their body, imagining themselves as being surrounded by a clear, violet aura of light. Then have them see in their mind's eye that this amethyst also includes the light of the black tourmaline and that it brings them strength, competency, ability, and the ability to realize whatever they set their mind to.

5. Now ask them to imagine that they have earthen-colored roots of light that flow from the bottoms of their feet deep into the earth, so that they have access to the power of the planet itself. Have them imagine that they are breathing in the power of the planet itself into their body so that they are mighty and capable of anything.

6. Now, have the person, while holding this sense of both peace and power, imagine a situation in which they feel anxious. Once they can see this in their mind's eye, have them become aware of any feelings in their body that occur as they maintain this image in their mind's eye. Continue breathing with long, deep, slow, and gentle breaths.

7. Ask them to now imagine that the amethyst light surrounds and dissipates this feeling in their body. This feeling leaves them with each slow exhale. Use your clear quartz crystal in your right hand to lift this feeling from the body and send it into Mother Earth where it is positively transformed, describing to the person what you are doing. If you feel this process getting stuck in any way, ask them if they are willing to release this feeling to you now so you can send it into the earth.

8. Once you have done that, have them breathe with long, deep breaths as if they flow in and out of their heart center as they relax with each breath.

9. Continue this process of the person seeing images that cause them anxiety and releasing them into the earth, followed by relaxing long, deep breaths in and out of their heart center.

10. When they are through, have them imagine filling their body with the rose-pink of the crystal in their heart center with every in-breath, relaxing with the out-breath. Continue until their body is completely filled with the pink light.

11. Next, have them silently repeat "I am capable and strong." Repeat this for three to seven minutes.

12. When you are done, remove the crystals in the opposite order in which you laid them, removing the rose quartz last.

I AM CAPABLE AND STRONG.

DISGUST AND CONTEMPT

Disgust or contempt can be a justified reaction to someone's behavior of which you disapprove. This is usually not a problem, as it passes quite easily, especially if you no longer are in the presence of that person and witnessing that behavior. If you find yourself thinking of that behavior and feeling disgusted or contemptuous, all you must do is drop those thoughts in favor of those more pleasant. It is a problem, however, when your disgust or contempt toward another is unfounded or based on them as a person rather than their behavior. Or it can be based on what you *imagine* to be their behavior. It is also a problem if you have these feelings about your own self, about your own essential self as a person.

Disgust and contempt of another person is quite often a defense mechanism to avoid your own feelings of inadequacy. Rather than experiencing these disturbing feelings of inadequacy, you may project them outwards onto another and then react with your disgust or contempt. If you feel contemptuous about yourself, it may be in reaction to your feelings of inadequacy that you don't project outwards but assimilate internally. It may be that you were disappointed in something that you did or didn't do, or you didn't act as you would have liked to. Then self-forgiveness is in order. However, deep-seated self-contempt or disgust most likely results from earlier wounding rather than just present behavior. Perhaps your parent or significant other, for example, treated you with contempt, so you treat yourself that way. Perhaps you were unloved, or abused, so rather than blame the parent or early caretaker, you treat yourself with contempt or disgust that you subconsciously think you deserve. These and other such reactions are common defense mechanisms.

The antidote to self-contempt or disgust is to substitute those feelings with those of adequacy and forgiveness, and to accept and approve of yourself just as you are. If you are projecting your own feelings of inadequacy onto another and then treating them with disgust or contempt, the best way to treat this is to discover your projection and experience the other person as they are. It is important to distinguish the difference between accepting yourself and others as they are and condoning misbehavior. They are two separate issues. You can think someone can or should change their behavior while at the same time accepting them as a person without the disgust and contempt. You can accept yourself as you are without disgust or contempt and still decide to change your actions for the better. It is also important to realize that deep-seated self-contempt or disgust cannot be treated in one or two treatments, as there are layers of wounding that need to be treated one by one. How to do this will be covered in the next chapter.

YOU CAN'T RECOGNIZE WHAT YOU DON'T ALSO HAVE WITHIN YOURSELF.

Here is a good crystal and stone healing to help experience yourself as competent and adequate so you will no longer need to project that onto another. It will help replace the contemptuous feelings that you carry within yourself with forgiveness, acceptance, and self-approval. This crystal healing is not only good for working with disgust and contempt, but also is applicable to many other emotionally painful conditions in which you have negative or disapproving experiences about your own self or others.

FORGIVENESS TECHNIQUE WITH CRYSTALS AND STONES

1. Sit upright in a chair or lay down flat on your back. Uncross your legs, hold your head straight forward, and hold your hands on your lap with your palms upright.
2. Surround your body with alternating amethyst and clear quartz crystals. Point their tips in toward the body. Start by placing the first amethyst over the head.
3. Now, place a clear quartz crystal above the amethyst that is over the top of your head. Point its tip downward toward your head. This will help open your crown energy center and channel higher awareness to you.

(Continued on next page)

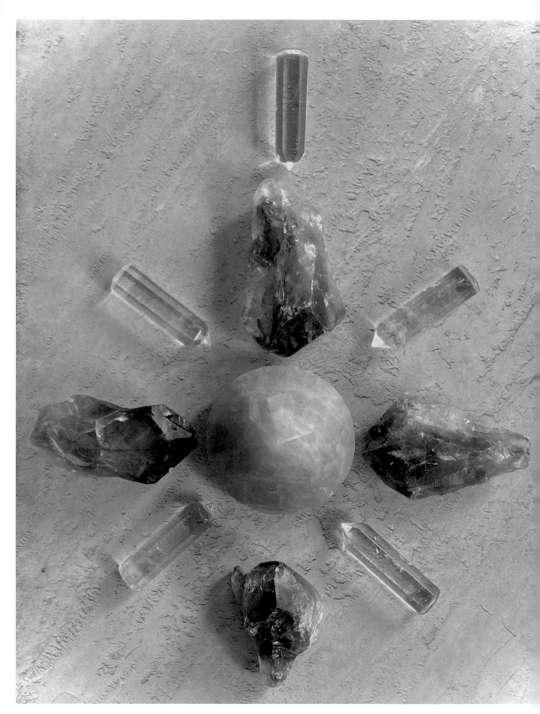

Crystal Layout for Forgiveness

4. Place a rose quartz on your heart center.

5. Now, hold another rose quartz between your two hands as you hold them together in prayer pose (as if you are praying). Bring your hands in prayer position up to the level of your heart center about 6 inches away. Point your fingers upward.

6. Now, close your eyes and focus on your breathing, breathing with long, deep, gentle breaths. Feel as if these breaths flow in and out of the rose quartz between your hands and from your heart center. With your eyes closed, bring your focus to your heart center. Relax your body with every out-breath. Especially relax any tension in the small of your back, your jaw, your stomach, or your chest.

7. Imagine that any feelings of contempt, disgust, or negative judgment of which you become aware leave your mind, heart, and body with every out-breath. As you do so, bring your focus back to your heart center.

8. Feel as if your heart glows with a gentle pink light. With every in-breath, imagine that light growing larger and larger until it fills your entire chest. Now imagine that the light gets larger and larger until your entire body is surrounded in a field of softly glowing pink light. Continue to breathe in and out of your heart center.

9. Now silently repeat these words: "I release all judgment toward others and myself." Release this judgment on your exhale. Then say "I accept others as they are." If you have someone specific that you have been disapproving of, repeat the words "I accept this person as they are." Then repeat to yourself: "I offer my forgiveness to this person." Then, "I forgive all others." Imagine that the aura of pink light surrounding you expands to include this other person or other people.

10. Finally, repeat the words "I forgive myself of all my shortcomings. I forgive others of their shortcomings." As you continue to repeat

(Continued on next page)

these words, imagine that you and any others upon which you focused are now surrounded together in a field of violet light.

11. Shift your focus back to your heart center while you are still surrounded in this gentle field of violet light. Breathe in love and forgiveness with every breath.

12. Remain in this violet field of light while breathing in love and forgiveness for at least ten minutes. There is no time limit in which you can remain in this state.

13. When you are through, while remaining in this state of forgiveness, imagine that a clear, bright light floods down from the heavens into your body, bringing you endless blessings as it fills you with its presence.

14. Once you have been blessed, open your eyes, maintaining this beautiful consciousness, and place the rose quartz between your hands down beside you. Now remove the crystals from your body in the reverse order in which you placed them.

15. See if you can maintain this consciousness as you go about your daily life.

16. Clear all the crystals and yourself. If you sense any residual negativity in the person you are working with, clear that from them also.

I FORGIVE MYSELF AND OTHERS.

I ACCEPT ALL OTHERS.

I ACCEPT MYSELF.

If you are helping another person with this process, as you repeat the instructions to them, use a clear quartz crystal in your right hand to remove any tension that you sense in their body and send it into the earth. As you instruct them to imagine the surrounding pink and violet aura, use an amethyst crystal to visualize surrounding their body with this light. As you instruct them to receive the clear light from above, use a clear crystal to visualize sending this light into their body, sweeping down from their head to their feet. Then visualize surrounding them in clear light. You can let them know that you are doing this to assist them, or if you determine that this will distract them from this meditation, just do it without telling them.

LONG-TERM APATHY AND EMOTIONAL WITHDRAWAL

Apathy is when you lack motivation to do anything that involves thinking or your emotions. Basically, you don't care what is going on around you or about anything in your life. In short, nothing in life interests you and you feel empty with no emotions at all.

Extreme apathy can be a condition related to Alzheimer's disease, forms of dementia, Parkinson's disease, stroke, head injury, problems with the area in the front of your brain, or a deep mental health problem. If you or another is suffering from this malady, a medical health professional should be consulted. You can still do your crystal emotional healing along with this other professional help.

Apathy may also be a sign of impending suicide, so before your treat anyone for this, you should determine if they have suicidal ideation, and if so, report it to a professional or the suicide hotline. Likewise, if you are feeling suicidal, have a talk with someone at the suicide prevention hotline.

Although they can seem quite similar, apathy is different from depression. Feeling withdrawn about life is common to both depression and apathy. It is also different than sadness. Sadness is emotional. Apathy is not. When apathetic, you don't feel any sense of motivation, you don't care about your problems, you don't want to meet new people or plan any activities, and nothing makes you excited or happy. Apathy depletes you energetically, robbing you of the desire to make any effort in life at all.

If not a medical issue, apathy is a suppression of emotions or a reaction to extreme anxiety. Apathy can be a dissociated state in reaction to being stuck in a life situation in which your needs are not being met. It can be used to indirectly construct a boundary when you cannot use your natural anger response, perhaps because you don't feel safe or the repercussions to your anger are judged to be too risky. In short, it is a coping mechanism that is not only designed to protect you, but to subtly strike out at people. (That is why people often respond with anger to someone who acts with apathy and withdrawal.)

Apathy and withdrawal can also be a response to the feeling that you will suffer extreme punishment or risk the loss of love from someone important to you. This sense of risk may be related to a recent life situation or can be a response to early childhood wounding.

If it is an emotional reaction to early wounding, it can take many sessions to reveal the deep layers of emotional suppression and correct the apathetic emotional reactions. If it is a more recent emotional response, you can help correct this in only one or a few treatments.

This crystal meditation can be used to help release the anger and its emotional suppression so that the apathetic response is no longer needed. It can help someone feel safe enough to develop a healthy anger response and resume normal relationships and an active, involved life.

> **APATHY IS THE OPPOSITE SIDE OF ANGER.**
> **THEY ARE TWO SIDES OF THE SAME COIN.**

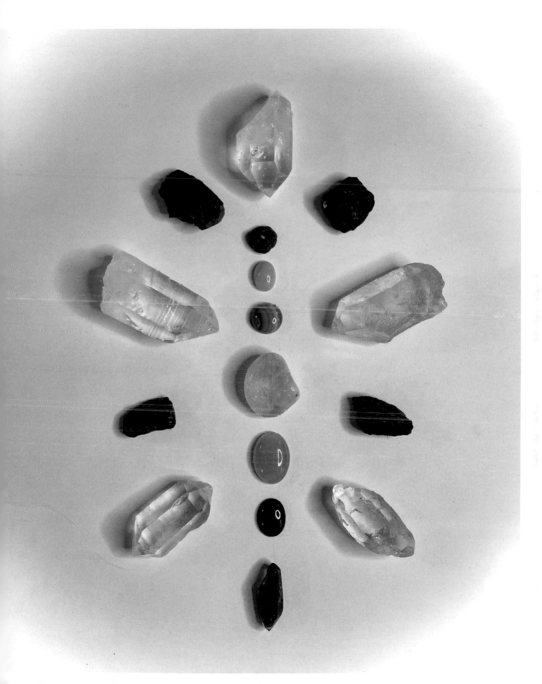

Crystal Layout to Relieve Apathy and Emotional Withdrawal

CRYSTAL AND STONE MEDITATION TO RELIEVE APATHY

1. Lay down on your back with your head forward, your legs uncrossed, and your hands down beside you with their palms upward.

2. Surround the body with alternating black tourmaline and clear quartz. You can also use black agate or another black stone. Say to the person, "These stones are creating a protective barrier around you so that you are strong and safe."

3. Place a red garnet hear the base of the spine, a yellow jade about 3 inches below the belly button, and a yellow citrine about 2 inches above the belly button. Say to the person, "These stones will bring you strength of will and strength of mind."

4. Place a green malachite on the heart center. If you don't have green malachite, place a green calcite on the heart center. Say to the person, "This stone will bring you back to yourself, and your heart will be safe to open."

5. Next, lay a royal blue azurite or lapis on the third eye point and a turquoise on the throat center. Say to the person, "This royal blue stone on your third eye will help reveal your innate wisdom and insight. This turquoise stone will help you feel safe and able to express yourself."

6. Place a clear quartz or Herkimer diamond in each upward-facing palm. Say to the person, "These crystals will help you feel capable, strong, and able to resist absorbing any negative emotion or judgment that is being sent to you."

7. Next, have the person breathe with long, deep breaths, imagining that the breath enters through the nurturing green malachite and their heart center and out through the yellow citrine on their abdomen. On the next breath cycle, have the person imagine that the breath is flowing in through the citrine and their abdomen, and out through the yellow jade on their belly. On the third breath cycle,

have the person imagine that their breath is flowing in through the yellow jade and their belly and out through the red garnet and the base of their spine. On the fourth breath cycle, imagine the breath flowing in through the red garnet and the base of their spine, up their body, and out through the green malachite and their heart center. Continue this four-part breath cycle for at least ten minutes, making sure that the person is not hyperventilating. Encourage the person to continue this breathing cycle, saying to them, "You are gathering strength with every breath."

8. Once the person has done this breath cycle for at least ten minutes, ask them to silently repeat: "I am strong." "I am okay as I am." "I am naturally powerful." Do this for at least three minutes.

9. Now, ask the person if there is anyone or a group of people that they feel anger toward. If they cannot think of anyone, ask them, "If you could be angry with someone or a group of people, who would they be?" (This may make it safer for them to feel angry with someone to whom they haven't felt safe expressing anger.)

10. If they can't imagine this, ask them the question, "Who do you *not* feel safe being angry with?" If they can't answer this, ask them; "If you imagine *not* feeling safe expressing your anger at someone, who would that person or those people be?"

11. If they still can't name a person or people with whom they *imagine* feeling anger, ask them to repeat these words: "It is safe to be angry. I am not a bad person when I am angry." Repeat these words for about three minutes.

12. Next, again repeat the questions, "If you could be angry with someone, who would it be?" and "If you could imagine feeling angry with someone, who would it be?"

13. Next, ask them to squeeze the clear quartz crystals in their hands as they answer the question, "If I could be angry, what would I like to

(Continued on next page)

say?" If they can't come up with a response, ask them if they would be willing to pretend to be angry and then ask them, "Pretending to be angry, what would you say?" Have them continue to squeeze the clear quartz crystals in their hands. Continue this until they have finished saying what they would like to.

14. If the person shows any sadness or other associated emotion, ask them to express in words what they are feeling. Let them know it is okay to feel this way.

15. When you are through, ask them to repeat the words, "I am strong and safe. It is okay to express myself." They can repeat these words as needed during the day.

16. Remove the crystals in the reverse order in which you placed them. Clear the other person by sweeping down their body with your clear quartz crystal from head to toe. Clear yourself as well. Then clear your crystals.

IT IS SAFE TO EXPRESS MYSELF.

GRIEF

Grief is incredibly painful. It is also part of a natural healing process. It is important to know that grief is a process through which you travel. Moving through the grief process is traveling the road to healing. If affects you emotionally, spiritually, physically, and mentally. It is both a natural response to losing someone or losing something important in your life like a loss of a profession.

Grief isn't the same for everyone, nor does it always take place in the same progression of anger, depression, bargaining, and acceptance. Though there are similarities between people who are grieving, ultimately it is an intensely personal, individual experience.

When grieving, it can be a physical shock as well as an emotional shock. It's important when grieving to continue eating, hydrating yourself, and sleeping. Be compassionate with yourself, allowing the process to unfold naturally. It cannot be forced, nor can you just "get over it." Nor is there any right or wrong amount of time that grief should take. The feelings of grief may come and go, but ultimately it is not a process that can be controlled. During the grieving process, you may feel tired, unable to concentrate, unbearably sad, angry, relieved, and depressed. You may be crying one moment only to laugh at something you remember about that person you have lost. The best way to heal grief is to let it unfold as it will and to be gentle with yourself.

The healing work we do with grief, then, is not to try to get over it, or remove it, but instead to honor what was lost and hold it in the psyche with gentleness and respect. The best way that you can work to help heal another's grief is to listen to whatever that person wants to share. Let them know that they can say anything to you and that they don't have to worry about your reactions. You are here to assist them through *their process,* that you have no agenda or opinions. Resist giving unsolicited advice or telling them that you know how they are feeling. You don't know exactly how they are feeling because everyone's process is different. They won't hear you anyway if it is unsolicited. Anytime that you want to share your thoughts, ask them first if it would be alright to share your thoughts with them. Be supportive, no matter how long it takes.

THERE IS NO RIGHT OR WRONG WAY TO GRIEVE.

Besides encouraging the person whom you are assisting through the grieving process to express themselves freely with you, an honoring ceremony can offer powerful healing help. The following is an honoring ceremony that can be done for you or for the other who is grieving:

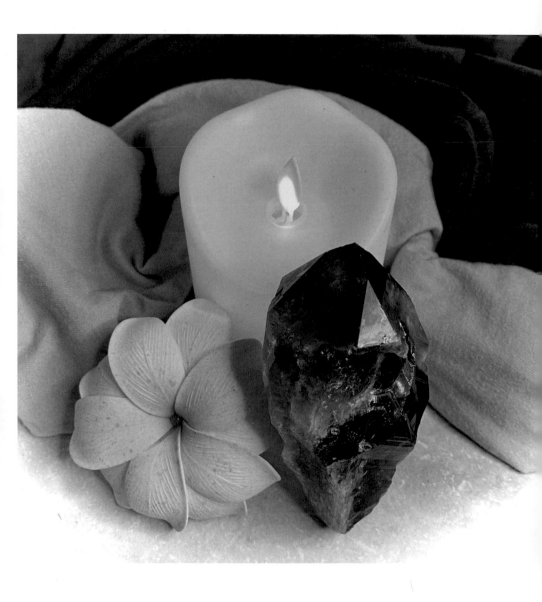

HONORING CEREMONY FOR GRIEF USING CRYSTALS

1. Select a meaningful location in which to have this ceremony or have it in your healing space that you have made special. If you have it in your healing space, darken the room with ambient lighting instead of bright lights. Surround the room with plants or flowers and have soft, meditative music playing. Have a special place for them to sit in the middle of the room that is comfortable. Opposite the seat, set up a small table. Dress up for the event in a way that acknowledges its importance. It is especially good to wear violet, pink, light green, or white. Avoid wearing black. Bring some flowers and two equal-sized candles to use during the ceremony. Bring an amethyst crystal that you can give to the person at the end of the ceremony. Have the person you are helping bring a wrapped picture of the person being honored that you unwrap and place in the center of the table.

2. Now have the person enter and sit down. Sit next to the person. If the picture of the person being honored is not set up on the table, have the person you are working with set up the picture.

3. Place a circle of alternating rose quartz and amethyst crystals around the person's chair with them in the center. Place a small amethyst crystal that you can give away in the person's left hand.

4. Now, have the person light one candle, saying "I invite your presence into this room with me." After a few moments, have them light the other candle, saying "I honor your life."

5. Now, have the person remember one thing that they loved about the person being honored. As they remember this, have them place one of the flowers in front of the picture. Next, have them remember another thing they loved about the person being honored. As they do so, place another flower in front of the picture.

(Continued on next page)

6. Have the person then remember something that the person being honored did for them or with them that made them especially happy. As they do so, place another flower on the table in front of the picture. Have them repeat this process, remembering something that the person did for them that made them happy and then placing a flower on the table.

7. Next, have the person remember an important event that they remember with happiness and place another flower. Have them next remember a beautiful quality that they remembered about the person being honored and place another flower in front of the picture.

8. Ask the person you are helping if there is anything that they would like to forgive about that person being honored, and if so, offer them forgiveness. Place another flower. Then ask the person you are helping if there is anything they would like to be forgiven for by the person being honored. If so, have them ask for it and then place another flower in front of the picture.

9. Now, have the person you are helping place the amethyst crystal that they have been holding in front of the picture of the person being honored. As they do so, have them repeat the words "I send to you beautiful violet light from this crystal and pray that you know happiness and joy through all eternity. May your soul be forever one with the Higher Spirit and may you dance forever in the field of joy and heavenly delight."

10. After these words, then say to the person you are helping, "Though the other is not in physical form, know that you are never separate, that you are joined in love through all eternity." After these words, have the person you are helping sit with palms upward in their lap as you circle them clockwise three times with the amethyst crystal from the table saying, "I bring you joy. I bring you love. I bring you peace." Say it three times, once with every circle.

11. Then, give the amethyst crystal to the person, letting them know that they can keep it in remembrance of this ceremony.

12. When the person is ready, have them close the ceremony by blowing out the candles. Remove the crystals surrounding them, placing them under the table and covering them. Give the other person the flowers from the ceremony. Take the picture from the table and wrap it again. Then hand the wrapped picture to the person with whom you are doing the ceremony.

13. Be sure that the person you are doing the ceremony with is grounded enough to leave. You can give them some water and use your crystals to ground them into the earth. Tell them to put the amethyst crystal in a special place and let them know that whenever they want to remember this ceremony, they have only to hold the crystal with eyes closed.

14. At no time should you rush through the ceremony or hurry their remembrances. Let them know it is okay for them to cry or express any emotion.

15. Once they have left, turn off the music and use the smoke of sage, cedar, or any herb that you feel rapport with to clear the room and then yourself.

Though this ceremony is simple, it can be quite profound. You can do it more than once with the person. At first, it may be too difficult to do. If not, you can do it just once, or do it once a week. Then as the person moves through their grief, they may want to do it once a month, and then only special times during the year.

GRIEF IS A MANIFESTATION OF LOVE.

FEAR

Fear is an emotional response caused by the belief that something or someone is dangerous, painful, or threatening. Fear can be based on real events or imaginary events. It can be based on events in the present or those that happened in the past. Whether based on what is actually real or what you are just afraid might happen in the future, the fear itself is real. It is a core human response that usually engenders the response of flight, fight, freeze, or appeasement. When you are fearful, it affects more than your emotions. Physically, adrenaline, cortisol, and other hormones are released into the brain and body. Your breathing becomes rapid and your heart rate and blood pressure increase. Blood flows away from your heart and into your limbs in preparation for flight or fight. These responses may happen both short and long term. Whether based on imagination or actual events, long or short term, fear robs you of your strength and enjoyment of life.

A particularly debilitating type of fear is phobia. Fear of heights, social situations, open spaces, enclosed spaces, fear of snakes, insects, or dogs are some usual phobias. If the person you are working with is suffering from phobia, it is good to refer them to a mental health professional who can work with desensitization and other therapeutic techniques. You can assist, however, by using your crystals and stones to help yourself or the other person to develop a sense of protective strength.

The ultimate fear for most people is the fear of death, of losing your own individuality, of losing your own existence. To work with this basic fear, it is helpful to help the person experience the reality of themselves beyond the physical body. Sometimes dreamwork can help, pointing out that your dream self seems as real as your physical self whether you are in a dream state or awake. You can also point out that even though nothing remains the same with our body, thoughts, or feelings, that even in the face of this constant change, we have a sense of ourselves that is permanent and unchanging.

The Ultimate Guide to Emotional Healing with Crystals & Stones

> **OUR ESSENTIAL SELF NEVER CHANGES.**
> **WE EXIST BEYOND THE PHYSICAL BODY.**

The following crystal and stone technique will help bring the fire element to the subtle body, strengthen the subtle and physical nervous system depletion, and help build a sense of protection and strength to combat fear.

CRYSTAL AND STONE TECHNIQUE FOR STRENGTH AGAINST FEAR

1. Lay down on your back or sit upright on a straight-backed chair. Uncross your legs and arms and face your head forward.
2. Surround your body with alternating yellow jade, yellow citrine, or other yellow crystals, and gold tiger eye. Place a red garnet or other red crystal at the base of your spine. Place a yellow citrine on your abdomen about 2 inches above your belly button. Place a clear quartz crystal over your heart chakra with its tip pointing upward. This will help shield the heart from absorbing attack or negative energy while keeping it open and active. Hold a clear quartz crystal in each hand. If it is single terminated, point the tip upward toward the arm so that it channels its energy into the subtle body.
3. Place a circle of clear quartz crystals about six inches beyond the circle of yellow and gold tiger eye crystals, so that you are surrounded with a double circle. Point their tips outward. This circle of clear quartz will help bring protection while the inner circle of crystals brings strength and the fire element.
4. Once these crystals and stones are set around the body, close your eyes. Imagine that you are surrounded with an orb of golden light.

(Continued on next page)

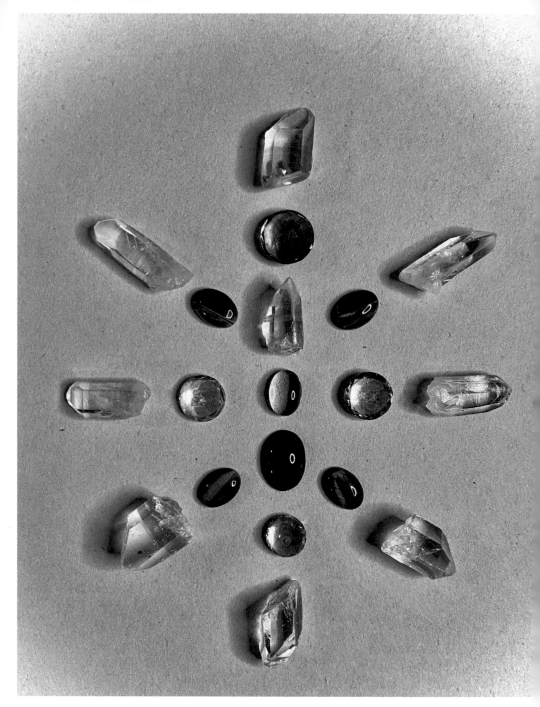

Crystal Layout for Strength Against Fear

Now, imagine that this golden light is absorbed through your skin until your body is filled with golden light. As this golden light fills your body, you feel more and more powerful, filled with the strength of firelight and the power of the sun. Silently repeat these words to yourself for at least three minutes: "I am filled with the life force energy of the universe. I am limitless. I am strong. I am beyond all fear."

5. Now shift your attention to the yellow crystal on your abdomen. Imagine that every in-breath brings its golden fire into your abdomen and belly. Imagine that your in-breath flows into your abdomen and that your out-breath flows out of your belly. Next, imagine that your in-breath flows in through your belly and out through your abdomen. Continue for three minutes. Imagine that you fill with power with every breath.

6. Next, imagine that your heart energy center in the middle of your chest now glows with a bright, clear light. With every in-breath, it gets brighter and brighter until it completely fills your body with clear, white light. Imagine that your breath now flows in and out through your heart energy center. Silently repeat these words to yourself for at least three minutes: "My love conquers all fear. I am safe and protected."

7. When you are through, continue breathing in and out of your heart energy center, releasing any tension that you may feel in your body with every out-breath and allowing the energy of this meditation to be completely absorbed into your body, mind, and being.

8. When you are through, open your eyes and then slowly remove all of the crystals on and around your body in the reverse order in which you placed them. Clear yourself and your crystals. If you are working with someone else, clear them, as well.

I AM SAFE AND PROTECTED.
I EMBODY THE LIFE FORCE OF THE UNIVERSE.

SADNESS

Sadness is a natural reaction to loss generally characterized by feelings of grief, helplessness, disappointment or sorrow, and a low mood. Someone feeling sad usually becomes withdrawn, increasingly quiet, or in extreme cases, completely silent. Because these forms of sadness contain elements of other forms of emotional distress, there is no one way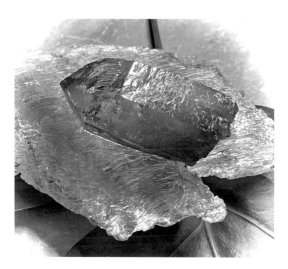

to treat sadness. We may find that the best way to treat sadness, for example, is to relieve the associated apathy or honor the grieving feelings associated with loss and hopelessness. Or we may need to explore and reexperience childhood wounds in the past that make us sad in the present.

Some forms of sadness do not necessarily have to do with loss or disappointment. Sometimes they may be poignant expressions of love and, thus, a pleasant experience. For example, you may feel poignant expression when you experience something special like exceptional kindness, or when you fondly remember a special person in the past. It can also be a response to love, especially if it reminds you of what you lost as children, or of people who you have lost in your life. It can also be in response to the openness and vulnerability that you experience in love and arousal, or a response to an experience of great beauty. These expressions of sadness are pleasant so do not need healing. If anything, they need honoring.

Methods to work with some of the underlying causes of painful sadness like loss and grief have been given to you earlier. Another good way to work with sadness, however, is to help bring a sense of connection

The Ultimate Guide to Emotional Healing with Crystals & Stones

with the healing and life-giving qualities of nature. When you are connected with nature, you can easily find a sense of timeless joy, growth, and nurturing acceptance that will help counter sadness. Nature can bring you into the presence of deep peace and healing to counter any emotional wounding or pain. This crystal and stone method is designed to connect you with the healing qualities of nature to help uplift your sadness, and to help bring you a sense of nurturing perspective.

CONNECTING WITH NATURE TO HEAL SADNESS

It is wonderful to do this crystal healing meditation outside in a natural setting if possible. If not, have your healing environment include plants and flowers and, if it is not cold, have the windows open to bring in the sunlight and gentle breezes of the outdoors. If you do this meditative technique outside, it is best to be done on green grass in a clearing where the ground is flat. Be sure that the person being healed is warm and comfortable. You may bring a light blanket and pillow that they can use. Before doing this healing, gather some flowers that you can place around the body during this healing meditation.

1. Whether you are outside or inside, have the person lie on their back with their legs uncrossed and their arms by their sides with their palms facing upward.

2. Start by placing a rose quartz or pink tourmaline on their heart energy center in the middle of their chest. If it is terminated, point its tip upward. Have them imagine their breath flowing in and out from the heart center, gathering a feeling of love into the heart center with every in-breath. Release any tension or negative feeling with the out-breath. Have them imagine the tension flowing down their body and out of their feet to enter Mother Earth, where it is

(Continued on next page)

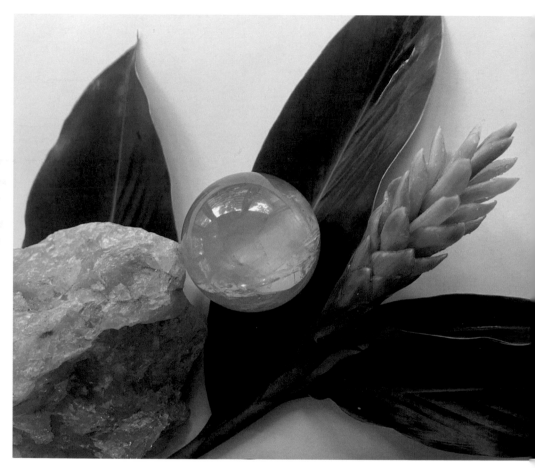

Rose Quartz with Nature

transmuted into positivity. Have them imagine the love flowing into their heart energy center as a beautiful, soft pink light. Then imagine the negative feeling as a gray light that transforms to a peaceful, soft green as it is transmuted. Do this for at least three minutes.

3. Now, place a flower over their crown, then circle clockwise to place two more flowers on the right side of their body, one below their feet, and another two at the right side of their body. As you do this, say, "The spirits of nature are blessing you with peace, joy, and abundance." If you have more flowers than this, you can use as many as you'd like to circle their body, repeating these words as you lay down each flower. If their eyes are closed, let the person know what color and type of flower you are using, saying words like, "I am laying this beautiful pink rose next to you" or "I am placing this white lily or yellow sunflower next to you." Then relay the blessing.

4. Next, outside the ring of flowers, surround their body with four, six, or eight alternating amethyst and green calcite crystals, starting with the amethyst over the crown, letting the person know what crystals you are using as you lay them down. As you lay down each crystal, say the words, "I am laying this amethyst over your head to bring you the peace of higher awareness and all healing, mind, body and spirit." Then "I am laying this gentle, light, green calcite to bring you the joyful, nurturing, life energy of the flowers, plants, trees, and all of nature." Continue in this manner until you have laid all the crystals around their body.

5. Now, place a green crystal or stone in each of their hands, saying "I lay this gentle, soft, green crystal in your hand so that nature's peace and healing can flow into your body, mind, and spirit."

6. Finally, place a smoky quartz beneath their feet at the outside of the circle of crystals and flowers. Point its tip downward into the earth.

(Continued on next page)

Say, "I have placed a soft brown smoky quartz beneath your feet so that you are rooted within the creative life force of Mother Earth." Have them imagine that the roots extend more and more into the earth with every out-breath.

7. Once all the flowers and crystals are placed, as their eyes remain closed, have them breathe with long, deep, full breaths that are gentle with no strain. Say to them, "With every in-breath, imagine that the joyful peace of Mother Earth flows through your heart energy center in the middle of your chest. Relax any tension that you feel in your body with the out-breath. With every in-breath, silently repeat to yourself, "I am held in the joyful, loving arms of Mother Earth." Remain in this state for ten minutes or longer.

8. When through, have them open their eyes as you carefully remove the crystals and flowers one by one in the reverse order in which you placed them. Give them the flowers to keep as a reminder of this meditation.

I AM GENTLY HELD IN THE LOVING ARMS OF MOTHER EARTH.

ENVY AND JEALOUSY

Jealousy and envy are unpleasant emotions for yourself as well as others who interact with you. Though people tend to use these terms synonymously, they aren't. They both involve feelings of "less than," that you want something that someone else has that you don't. However, they are somewhat different. Being a mixture of both admiration and dissatisfaction, envy is less hostile and usually thought to be less negative than jealousy. It is not necessarily spiteful or mean and can also be used as a compliment. In contrast, when you feel jealous, you generally feel some degree of threat, protectiveness, and hostility. Jealousy involves feeling bitter or resentful that someone has something that you want. It is centered more on the person than the thing that you desire.

When you are jealous, it often brings up negative feelings about yourself, that you "aren't enough" or somehow deficient. You fall short in your estimation. Because of this, you feel some degree of hostility toward the person of whom you are jealous. The other person may then feel a sense of disquiet around you as they sense your jealousy. They may return your hostility with their own hostile feelings. When you are jealous, you drive people away from you. This, in turn, makes your jealousy worse because you then seem to have even less of what the other person has that you don't. It can be a vicious circle.

Jealousy, especially intense and reoccurring jealousy that interferes with your relationships and daily living, can be a symptom of an anxious attachment style that stems the early childhood relationship with your parents in which you feared abandonment, felt underappreciated, experienced inconstant care or a chaotic or scary environment. Anxious attachment causes you to obsess over whether someone likes you, wants you, or is thinking about you. If you think that they don't, which is usually the case of someone with this attachment disorder, your negative feelings about yourself take over, and you withdraw, sometimes so much that you can become completely paralyzed in life, unable to function normally. Because of your intense fear of rejection, you push people away before they can abandon you like you think they are going to eventually do. You have trouble trusting people. This all can support constant states of jealousy.

FOCUS ON WHAT *IS* RATHER THAN WHAT *IS NOT*.

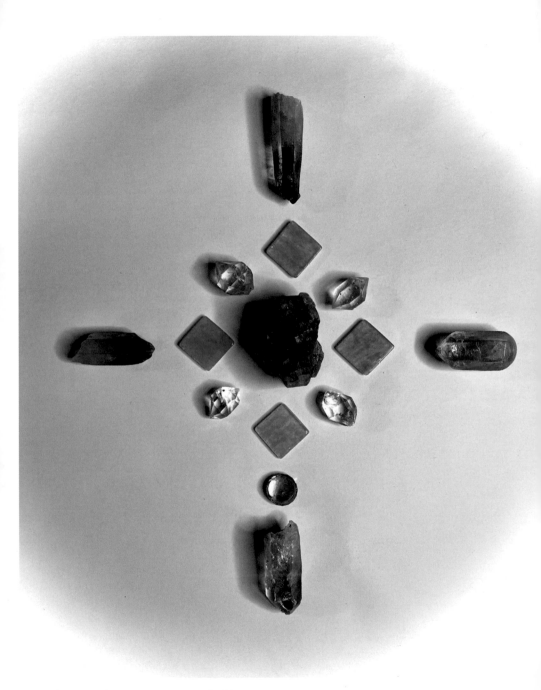

Crystal Layout for a Secure Sense of Self

To heal yourself of jealousy, you must change your focus, to concentrate on your own strengths, on what you do have, rather than what you think you lack or don't have. You need to overcome your insecurity and your lack of self-confidence that stem from your early childhood experience and instead learn to experience your own value. You need to learn that you are enough just as you are, that there is nothing lacking about you, that you are just as valuable a human being as anyone else. In short, to heal jealousy, especially jealousy stemming from an anxious attachment disorder, you must change your belief systems about yourself and other people and develop your sense of self-esteem. You need to feel worthy just as you are.

CRYSTAL AND STONE TECHNIQUE TO DEVELOP A SECURE SENSE OF SELF

1. Lie on your back with your legs uncrossed, your head forward, and your arms by your side, palm facing upward in receptive position.
2. Place a pink tourmaline or rose quartz on the heart center in the middle of the chest. Surround the pink crystal with four gentle green calcites or other green crystals to amplify the heart opening effects of the pink crystal. Place one green crystal above and touching the rose quartz or pink tourmaline. Place another to the right and touching the pink crystal. Place another green crystal below and touching the pink crystal on the heart center. Place the fourth green crystal to the left and touching the pink crystal.
3. Now, place small clear crystals or Herkimer diamonds around the pink tourmaline or pink crystal on the heart center, one in between each of the green crystals so that you have surrounded the center pink crystal with eight alternating green and clear crystals. This will open the heart center, while bringing a sense of protection.

(Continued on next page)

4. Breathe with slow and deep breaths, feeling as if each in-breath and out-breath flows in and out of the heart center in the middle of your chest. With each in-breath, silently say to yourself, "It is safe to love. It is safe to feel vulnerable." As you silently repeat these words, relax your body on every out-breath. Do this for at least three minutes.

5. As you breathe in and out of your heart energy center, allow any tears, fear, anger, or any other negative emotion to arise, naming it as it does. For example, if tears or sadness arise, say "I feel tearful or I feel sad." Allow these feelings to arise, and then on the out-breath, imagine them flowing out of you into the earth where they are accepted into the arms of Mother Earth where they are healed. Continue for another three minutes or until you feel that you are through.

6. As you let these feelings be released, bring your attention back to your heart center and feel as if your breath flows in and out of it. Do this for three minutes.

7. Now place four, six, or eight amethysts in a circle around the body; one above the head; one, two, or three on the right side; one below; and one, two, or three on the left side of the body. In your mind's eye, see yourself as surrounded with violet light. Then with every in-breath, imagine it flowing in through your skin to fill your body with its healing light. Do this for another three minutes.

8. Place a yellow citrine on your belly button. If it is terminated, point the tip upward. Silently say to yourself, "I am joyful. I am happy. I am safe. I am protected from all that I fear." Silently repeat these words for another three minutes.

9. Place a pink tourmaline, rose quartz, or other pink crystal in each upward-facing hand. As you do, silently say to yourself, "I am filled with love." Silently repeat these words for three minutes.

10. Now that you are resting in the pink glow of love, filled with the violet light of healing and acceptance, think of something about

yourself that you like. Say what it is silently or out loud. If you can't think of a positive quality about yourself, say, "If I had a positive quality, what would it be?" or "If I could think of a positive quality about myself, what would it be?" Continue to think of positive qualities about yourself for at least three minutes.

11. Next, think of something that you think that you do well. Say what it is silently or out loud. If you cannot think of anything that you do well, say to yourself: "If I could imagine myself doing something well, what would it be?" Continue to think of what you do well or could imagine yourself doing well for three minutes.

12. After that, think of more positive qualities about yourself, or if you cannot, say: "If I could imagine a positive quality about myself, what would it be?" Do this for another three minutes.

13. Finally, squeezing the pink crystals that you have in each hand, silently repeat the words "I believe in myself. I am okay just as I am. I am worthy of love." Do this for at least three minutes.

14. When you are through, bring your attention back to your heart center in the middle of your chest, feeling as if your breathing flows in and out of it. Do this for another three minutes.

15. When you are through, remove the crystals in the reverse order in which you placed them. When you are through, open your eyes. Clear yourself and all the crystals. If you are helping someone else with this process, clear yourself, as well.

16. Silently repeat the words, "I believe in myself. I am okay just as I am, and I am worthy of love" as you go about your day.

THERE IS NO SUCH THING AS A PERFECT PERSON.

SHYNESS OR FEAR OF REJECTION

A little shyness is quite usual and nothing to be concerned about. If it is so much that it negatively affects your social life, however, then it is a problem. This is the type of social anxiety that is of concern, and the type you will find yourself working with to heal.

Shyness is an error in reasoning in which you worry people will notice and negatively judge your mistakes or quirks. Rather than asserting your individuality, if you are shy, you tend to avoid being noticed or bringing attention to yourself. You might feel as if all eyes are on you when you enter a room, although that is seldom the case unless you are doing something unusual or looking odd. When you are shy, suffering from the spotlight effect, it means that you tend to assume that your mistakes and personal flaws that you think you have stand out clearly to others, and so, if they notice you, you will be rejected. Shyness, then, is quite often related to a lack of confidence in yourself. This lack of self-confidence is seldom related to your abilities or personal traits. Instead, it is based on what you consciously or unconsciously think about yourself. People who are shy feel nervous, bashful, timid, or insecure and notice physical sensations like blushing, feeling speechless, or breathless. They may feel shaky inside when around other people. When people know what to expect, or are among familiar people or in familiar situations, they are likely to feel less shy.

I AM THE LIGHT OF THE HIGHER SPIRIT.

Shyness is not a bad thing, only when it becomes overwhelming enough that you avoid social situations entirely because they are just too anxiety-provoking. In fact, shyness, if it's not debilitating, can even be a gift. A shy person may be more sensitive to people's feelings, and if so, is especially caring. Since they often prefer listening to talking, they can be good friends and especially supportive.

Shyness shouldn't be confused with introversion. When you are an introvert, you may be similarly quiet in social situations, but you don't have trouble socializing. It is, instead, that you aren't socializing because you aren't in the mood, or you prefer your own company. You choose to spend time alone because you require quite a bit of solitude. Unlike a shy person, you don't feel uncomfortable around people because you fear rejection or disapproval or criticism, only that you aren't in the mood at the time.

The roots of debilitating shyness, then, are like those of jealousy and anxiety. They are all responses to anxiety and a lack of confidence in yourself. When you work with shyness, you can use the crystal healing techniques that have been given here for anxiety and confidence. You can also use this emotional healing technique:

USING CRYSTALS TO REDUCE SHYNESS AND SOCIAL ANXIETY

1. Sit upright in a straight-backed chair or lie down on your back.
2. Surround yourself with an even number of alternating clear quartz and amethyst crystals with their tips pointing in toward your body. You can start with either an amethyst or clear quartz over your crown, and then lay the alternating crystals around your body in a clockwise circle.
3. Place a lapis stone or royal blue crystal over your third eye. If you are sitting up, wear the royal blue crystal on a headband. Place a rose quartz or pink crystal over your heart energy center in the middle of your chest. If you are sitting up, you can wear a rose quartz pendant on a 24-inch chain or a chain that places the crystal over the heart

(Continued on next page)

Healing Techniques for Common Emotional Upsets

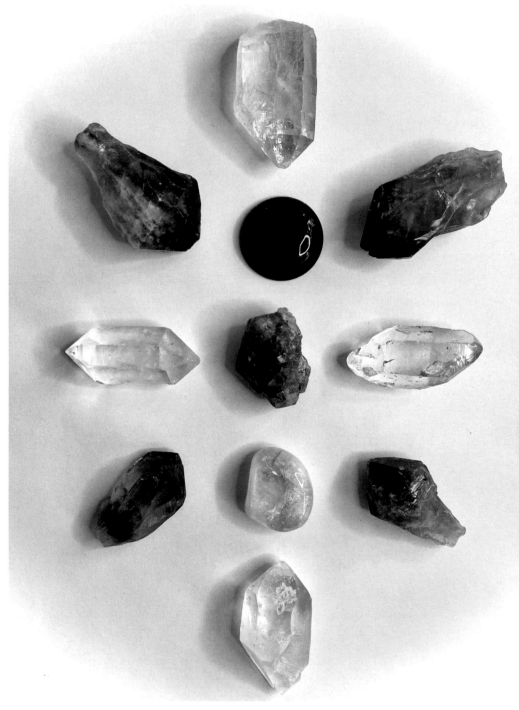

Crystal Layout to Reduce Shyness and Social Anxiety

center. Hold an empowering clear quartz crystal in each hand with its tip pointing in toward your arm.

4. Place a light-yellow citrine or yellow jade on your belly button. If you are sitting up, you can tuck it into a belt.

5. Close your eyes and feel as if you are breathing in and out of your heart energy center. Imagine that you fill with loving energy with every in-breath. Relax your body with every out-breath.

6. When you feel centered into yourself, imagine yourself in a social situation or with a person with whom you feel shy. When you have this picture clearly in your mind's eye, notice how your body is feeling. Notice if your breathing becomes more rapid, if your stomach tightens, if your jaw clenches, or any other sensation. As you notice each sensation, take a deep breath, and then exhale, imagining that this sensation releases.

7. As you continue to visualize yourself in the social situation, notice whether you are feeling fearful. If so, shift your attention to your belly and the yellow crystal. Breathe in through your belly and the yellow stone, feeling as if you are gathering the fear. Take the clear crystal in your right hand and circle clockwise around the fear that you feel in your belly. Then on your out-breath, release the fear. As you do that, imagine that the fear flows into the crystal. Then point your crystals to the ground and let the fear flow into the earth, where it is positively transmuted. Continue for at least three to ten minutes.

8. Now, as you continue to imagine yourself in the social situation or with the person with whom you are fearful, notice if you have any negative judgments about yourself. If you do, one by one, imagine that they flow into your clear quartz crystal, and again, point the crystal into the earth, imagining that these negative judgments or thoughts about yourself flow into the earth where

(Continued on next page)

Healing Techniques for Common Emotional Upsets

they are positively transmuted. Continue doing this for at least three to ten minutes or until you cease to experience any negative self-judgments.

9. Now, placing both of your hands in your lap, while still holding the clear quartz crystals, think of something that you like about yourself. When you find something that you like about yourself, imagine that that thought flows into the clear quartz crystal in your right hand. Then, still focusing on the positive thought, touch the tip of your right-hand crystal that contains the positive thought to your heart center in the middle of your chest. Inhale with a deep breath, and then as you let it out, imagine that that positive thought about yourself enters your heart center.

10. Continue thinking about positive things about yourself and sending them into your heart center with the crystal. If you cannot think of anything positive, *imagine* something that might be positive about yourself. See yourself as having this positive quality in your mind's eye, let it flow into the clear quartz crystal, and pass it into your heart center. Do this for at least three to ten minutes.

11. Now, imagine yourself in a social situation or with a person with whom you felt fearful. Imagine yourself in that situation glowing with loving, accepting energy and glowing bright light. Imagine yourself as being accepted by the other people in that social situation. See the others and you as being joined in a violet field of accepting and peaceful light. Do this for three minutes.

12. Once you are through, hold both hands with the crystals upward on your lap in a receptive position. Imagine that a clear light flows into your hands and flows upward to fill your entire body. With each inhale, allow more clear light to enter your body. Silently repeat: "I am perfect just as I am. I am strong. I am the light of the Higher Spirit." Repeat these words for at least three minutes. Continue repeating them as you go about your daily activities.

The Ultimate Guide to Emotional Healing with Crystals & Stones

I AM A VALUABLE PART OF SPIRIT'S CREATION.

SHAME

Shame makes you focus your attention inward where you view yourself in a negative light. Whereas guilt leads you to focus on what others think about you, or is connected to a concrete action, when you carry a sense of shame, you feel that there is something intrinsically wrong with you. Often resulting from early events when you felt humiliated, a sense of shame brings low self-esteem or depression. Shame makes you feel bad about yourself. You feel small, often wishing that you could just vanish. Shame can result from your sense of violating a behavioral norm. It brings uncertainty regarding how to fit in with external expectations and fundamental embarrassment about yourself. Because shame makes you disapprove of yourself, you feel that others will disapprove of you, as well.

Guilt and shame, which can be easily confused, are different though somewhat related. When you feel shame, you tend to view *yourself* in a negative light. In contrast, when feeling guilty, you tend to view *your actions* in a negative light. When feeling shameful, for example, you might tell yourself, "I am a terrible person." In contrast, when feeling guilty, you may tell yourself, "I never do anything right." In both cases, however, you negatively judge yourself. Guilt and shame often occur together to some extent. A sense of guilt can trigger a sense of shame. Both shame and guilt may merely be passing feelings, easily overcome by correcting your actions. However, they become debilitating when they reflect a fundamental and deep way that you feel about yourself.

When you are suffering from shame, you may avoid eye contact, maintain physical distance from people, or seem to be shrinking inside of yourself. When you feel shameful, you want to be hidden and alone. You

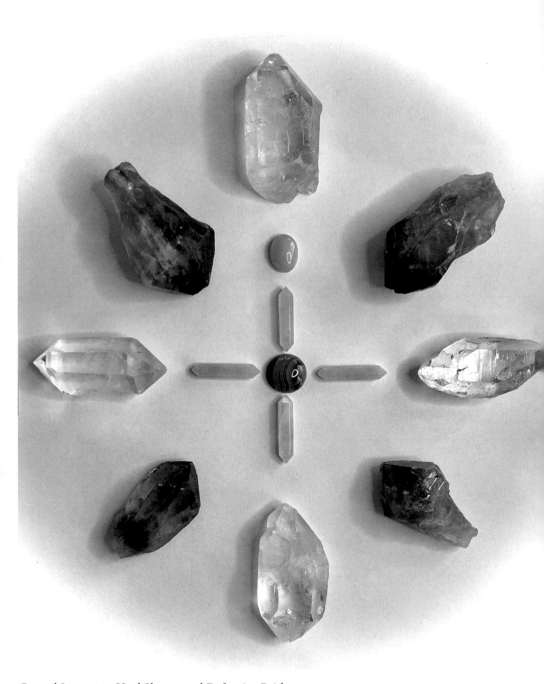

Crystal Layout to Heal Shame and Defensive Pride

don't want to be seen or heard. Shame sucks you into a heavy darkness in which you feel that you are "bad" or fundamentally broken.

Shame is also related to pride—not the pride based on success, but instead the pride by which you try to hide yourself. They are two sides of the same coin. Both keep you protected from feeling vulnerable. Trying to not feel vulnerable, you often run back and forth between pride and shame. When you feel shameful, you have the feeling that you aren't as good as anyone else, so you don't have to be vulnerable. When you feel prideful, you feel like you are better than everyone else, so you don't have to be vulnerable. However, they are both hiding places that keep you from real self-expression and interaction with others. Both are lonely. Because you can't know yourself, you cannot know other people.

To heal from shame, you must bring your shameful self to light instead of hiding yourself. It may be terrifying to receive help to heal from shame, as it involves revealing shameful feelings that may bring you the rejection that you fear. You may be afraid to find out that the shame you feel is deserved. When healing shame, then, you must learn to feel compassion for yourself, recognizing that everyone has flaws, that you are no different than anyone else . . . neither better nor worse.

CRYSTAL AND STONE TECHNIQUE TO HEAL SHAME AND DEFENSIVE PRIDE

1. Lay on your back with legs uncrossed and arms down by your sides, palms upward. Place a green malachite on your heart center. Surround it with four rose quartz crystals, one on top, one on the side, one on the bottom, and one on the other side. Point their tips in toward the green malachite. Place a small amethyst in between each rose quartz with their tips pointing outward. This crystal layout

(Continued on next page)

promotes the opening of the heart center to bring higher awareness and wisdom.

2. Surround the body with healing amethyst alternated with clear quartz crystals. Point the tips of the amethyst in toward the body to channel in a sense of safety, higher awareness, and healing. Point the tips of the clear quartz crystals outward to help reduce the tendency to hide and shrink into the self.

3. Hold a clear quartz crystal in each hand with the tips pointing up toward the hand. This will help bring energy into the body to help encourage a sense of self-empowerment.

4. Place a small turquoise on the throat energy center in the middle of the throat. This will help bring the ability to communicate the feelings that you have about yourself.

5. Begin to breathe with long, deep breaths imagining that the breaths flow in and out of your heart energy center. Relax your body with each out-breath. With every in-breath, imagine that you are allowing compassion and love to flow into your heart center. Do this for at least ten minutes.

6. Now, continuing to draw love and compassion for yourself into your heart center, imagine that you feel shame and let it release on your out-breath. Do this for at least ten minutes.

7. Give voice to any shameful feelings that you experience about yourself. If you cannot locate any shameful feelings, imagine that you have shameful feelings and say what they are. Release them on your out-breath. Continue for at least three minutes.

8. Notice any bodily sensations that arise for you as you relay these shameful feelings. If you cannot find any bodily sensations, imagine that you do and say what they are. Let them release with every out-breath. Continue this for at least three minutes.

9. Bring your breathing back to your heart center and imagine that the violet light surrounding you glows brighter and brighter with every

in-breath until you are completely surrounded in an orb of healing violet light. Relax on the out-breath.

10. Once you are filled with violet light, imagine that a bright, purple ray of light flows down through the top of your head, down through your body to completely fill it with purple light. Breathing in and out, imagine that you are floating within a field of violet light that extends outward farther than your eye can see.

11. With the vision of this violet light in your mind's eye, let yourself be filled with happiness, acceptance, compassion, and love with every breath you take.

12. Still within the violet healing field of light, silently repeat these words to yourself: "I deserve to be happy. I am a good person. I deserve love." Repeat these words to yourself for at least ten minutes. If your mind wanders, bring it first back to the violet light in your mind's eye, then continue repeating these words to yourself.

13. When you are through, imagine that the violet light in which you float begins to recede more and more so that it is eventually entirely within your body. Breath in wisdom and peace as this happens.

14. Let the light remain within your body as you remove the crystals in the reverse order in which you placed them. Leave the green malachite on your heart center and take three long, deep, peaceful breaths and imagine that they flow in and out of your heart center. With your attention remaining on your heart center, remove the green malachite crystal.

15. Open your eyes if someone has been laying the crystals on your body for you. See if you can retain this feeling of love and self-acceptance within you as you continue your day. Continue to silently repeat "I deserve to be happy. I am a good person. I deserve love" to yourself as you go about your days.

16. Clear your crystals, the room in which you did this process, and yourself. If you have been helping during this process, clear yourself also.

OBSESSION AND COMPULSION

Obsessive-Compulsive Disorder (OCD) is an anxiety-related psychological disorder in which you suffer from repetitive images or thoughts that are intrusive and unwanted. Accompanying this condition are ritualistic, repetitive behaviors that you believe or are compelled to do to hold these thoughts or images at bay or to make them easier to avoid. Ultimately, these behaviors are designed to manage anxiety. With the use of rituals or repetitive behaviors, your anxiety becomes less intrusive, and the sense of possible doom or disaster abates. Though healing OCD can be difficult and multifaceted, it basically involves helping you learn to tolerate the fear and uncertainty that feed your anxiety. While linked to anxiety with its accompanying cognitive and behavioral components, there are other biological factors that may also be the cause of OCD. Among these are the antibody response to infections, a response to a traumatic incident either in childhood or adulthood, basic brain physiology with abnormal activity or serotonin issues, or genetics. Some of the more usual obsessive compulsive behaviors, which are often exaggerated versions of worries that most people have at some time, include: frequent handwashing, excessive showering, bathing, or grooming with accompanying fear of contamination and of germs, obsessively checking doors or windows to be sure they are closed, obsessively checking appliances repeatedly to make sure they are turned off, counting in certain repetitive patterns, silently repeating words or phrases, arranging and rearranging objects, hoarding, rituals designed to ward off contact with superstitious objects, extreme perfectionism, fear of being responsible for something terrible happening or of harming others, fear of horrible images in the mind, fear of losing control, unwanted sexual thoughts and sexual obsessions, repeating activities in multiples or "safe" numbers, obsessively repeating routine activities like getting up and down from a chair.

The most common form of treatment for OCD is sensitivity training with exposure and response prevention. Neurofeedback, light therapy, acupuncture, exercise, and mindfulness meditation have also been shown to be helpful. It is best, however, to have someone who suffers from OCD consult a medical or psychiatric professional as you assist their healing process with the work that you do. The work you do should help the person suffering from OCD become more comfortable with their anxiety when exposed to what they fear. The anxiety healing already explained in this book is helpful for someone with OCD. You can also do the following healing:

HELPING WITH OBSESSIVE COMPULSIVE ANXIETY DISORDER

1. Be sure that your healing environment feels entirely safe for the one being healed. He or she should feel well protected.
2. Have the person sit upright in a straight-back chair. Sit opposite them with a small table in front of you. Have a large, clear crystal or crystal ball sitting upright on the table. Darken the room slightly, making sure that the person feels comfortable. Shine a light or candle into the crystal.
3. Surround their body with four, six, or eight alternating black tourmaline, or other black stones, and amethyst crystals, pointing their tips inward. As you lay the crystals in a clockwise position around the person being helped, let them know that the black stones will bring them complete protection from all fears and anything that might harm them. The amethyst crystals will bring a sense of peaceful awareness and healing. Have the person hold an amethyst in each hand with the tip pointing up toward the arm.

(Continued on next page)

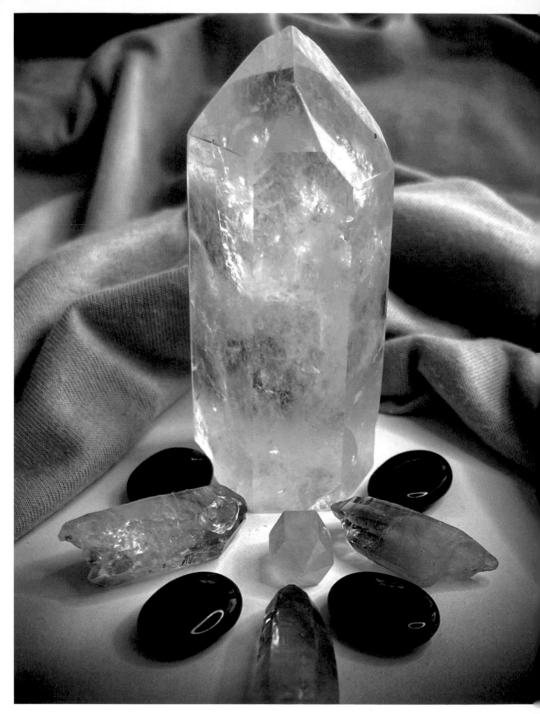

Crystals to Help with Obsessive/Compulsive Anxiety Disorder

4. Place a rose quartz on their heart center, or they may wear a rose quartz on a chain that rests it on their heart center.

5. Hold a clear quartz crystal in each of your hands. In your left receptive hand, point its tip up toward your arm. In your right transmitting hand, point the tip of the crystal outward toward your fingertips. Wear a royal blue lapis, sapphire, or other blue crystal on your third eye in the center of your forehead. Or wear lapis, sapphire, or other royal blue crystal earrings. This will help bring you insight and psychic awareness as you lead the person being healed in this process.

6. Have the person you are working with breathe in and out of their heart center, relaxing their body with every out-breath. With every in-breath, have them feel as if they are breathing in peace and protective calmness. Do this for at least three minutes or until they feel completely calm.

7. Now have them look into the crystal in front of them, noticing something interesting, or where they just feel drawn to look. Have them look at it more closely, noticing more detail. Keep leading them deeper into the crystal. Continue to lead them into the crystal until they lose their awareness of anything else. They may feel as if they are inside the crystal. At this point, their eyes may close. If they are still concentrated, that is okay. Let them know that they are completely safe inside the crystal.

8. Tell the other person that you are inside the crystal with them, to help them feel safe and secure.

9. Now, have them imagine something that makes them feel anxious. Guide them to completely feel their anxiety rather than trying to avoid it as they usually would. At the same time, guide them to continue breathing with long, slow breaths in and out of their heart center without gasping or hyperventilating.

(Continued on next page)

10. Have them notice where in their body they feel anxiety or fear. Have them continue to breathe in and out of their heart center with long, slow, easy breaths as they do this.

11. Have them notice if they have any thoughts about what they are feeling anxious about and tell you these thoughts aloud. After each thought, have them breathe in and out of their heart center with easy, slow breaths without gasping or straining in the least.

12. Once you have done these three steps, guide them to again imagine something anxiety-producing, again noticing where they feel it in their body along with their accompanying thoughts. Have them continue to breathe with long, slow, gentle breaths in and out of their heart center without gasping or straining.

13. Do this process three times or as many times as they feel comfortable doing. When you are through, have them continue to breathe in and out of their heart center as you guide them to imagine themselves inside the crystal, then outside of it, then see it get smaller and smaller until they can imagine it sitting in front of them.

14. Have them continue to breathe in and out of their heart center, relaxing their body on every out-breath and bringing in loving peace with every in-breath. Do this for at least three minutes or until they are completely relaxed.

15. When relaxed, have the other person open their eyes. Use your crystal in your right hand to clear them, sweeping their body from head to toe, down their arms, and out their fingertips. As you clear them with your crystal, have them exhale any tension that may remain within them, so they are totally clear. When you are through, clear all the crystals and yourself. Clear the room in which you did this process.

16. Remove the crystals from their body and from around them one by one in the opposite order in which you placed them.

The Ultimate Guide to Emotional Healing with Crystals & Stones

DEPRESSION

Depression is a painful mental and emotional disorder that affects how you feel, the way you think, and how you act. It may be characterized by feelings of sadness, a loss of appetite, changes in sleep or appetite, reduced energy or manic energy, inability to concentrate, or low self-esteem. People who are depressed may exhibit anxiety or apathy, guilt, irritability with angry outbursts or frustration, or have a persistent sense of hopelessness. Their sleep may be disrupted either by the inability to sleep, or excessive sleeping. They may experience sudden weight gain or weight loss. Also common is repeatedly going over the same thoughts in their head, or thoughts of suicide. They may experience a loss of interest in their normal activities or have sudden mood swings. Because depression exhibits so many characteristics, it is very difficult to work with, especially since someone who is depressed often holds onto the thought that there is nothing that can be done to help them and then resists any help at all.

Everyone has spells of feeling low or unhappy, but if it lasts more than a few days, or is persistent and deep, you are likely suffering from a mood disorder that calls for clinical diagnosis and is best handled with medical or psychiatric intervention. You can then augment their efforts with your crystal and stone healing help. If you have mild depression rather than a clinical depressive disorder, it may be characterized by simply experiencing a persistent low mood that can get better over time. It is common to feel depressed if you are stressed, grieving a loss or the death of a loved one, after having a baby, or if you are anxious because you are experiencing a difficult time in your life. You can also be depressed without an obvious reason. This milder type of depression does not usually take the intervention of a medical professional and can be treated by you.

Besides the healing work that you do with your crystals and stones, there are some other things that will help. First, since a depressed person tends to retreat from life, it helps to assist the person you are working with to set a life routine that they agree to follow. Because you are less focused on accomplishment and more on getting them out of their negative self-involvement, this routine can be simple. What is important is to follow it. Following this same idea, encourage the person you are working with to take on some responsibilities. Again, they can be simple. Perhaps they can volunteer twice a week at an animal shelter, work a couple days a week, babysit a few evenings a week, and so on. The focus isn't on what they do, only that they continue with the responsibilities they have chosen. It is important for someone who is depressed to stop drinking alcohol, avoid recreational drugs, and follow a healthy diet, all things that a depressed person may be indulging in, usually to mask the depressive symptoms. Since exercise helps reduce depressive symptoms, encourage the depressed person to set up an exercise program that they follow. Sunlight also helps alleviate depression, so encourage them to get out of the house and be in the sunlight. Morning walks in the sun are an excellent program to encourage. Other ways of working with depression that can help are positive self-talk, guided discovery, present moment awareness, and cognitive restructuring.

Here is a crystal healing practice that you can do to help with mild depression. It employs all four healing methods. You can do them with yourself as well as another person. It is easier to work with someone else, however, that can guide your process with the necessary degree of perspective that will allow them to make suggestions that are workable.

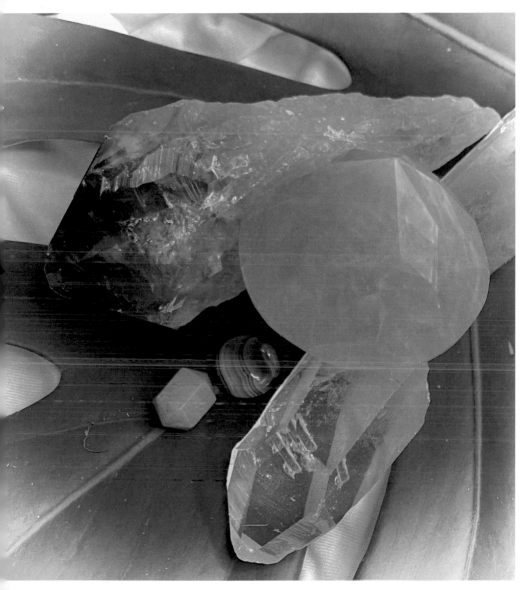

Amethyst, Rose and Clear Quartz, Malachite, and Green Aventurine for Depression Relief

USING CRYSTALS AND STONES TO HELP HEAL DEPRESSION

1. Create a safe, comfortable, and welcoming environment in which to do this healing process. Surround your room with rose quartz crystals, visualizing them as being connected with streams of rose-colored light. Have your room be filled with sunlight. If it isn't sunny outside your windows, you must be sure that they let in lots of light. Turn the lights on in your room to a comfortable brightness. Let them know that whatever they say to you is confidential and *you will not judge them whatever they say*. Fill your room with plants or flowers and inspiring pictures. If it is a warm, sunny day, you can do this healing outdoors on green grass surrounded by trees and other plants.

2. Wear pastel or white colors as you work with them. Also wear a rose quartz on your heart center, turquoise near your throat center, and lapis near your third eye. This will allow your heart to remain open and for you to hear the wisdom that comes from an open heart. The lapis will help bring insight, and the turquoise will help you find the words to express what you "see" during the session. (Generally, a pendant on a 24-inch chain will bring a crystal near your heart center, a 16- or 15-inch chain will lay it near your throat center, and earrings will bring the stones near your third eye unless you wear a headband.)

3. Invite the other person to lie down on their back in the center of the healing space with their legs uncrossed, their head forward, and their arms down by their sides, palms upward.

4. Lay a rose quartz, pink tourmaline, or other pink stone on their heart center, saying to them, "I am laying this gentle, loving crystal on your heart. Let its love enter your heart. May you be tender with yourself." Guide them at this time to feel as if their breath flows in and out of their heart center. With every in-breath, have them draw in the love and tender feeling of the pink crystal. With every out-breath,

let them relax their chest, stomach, small of their back, neck and shoulders, and jaw.

5. Using a clear quartz crystal in your right hand, sweep down their body, about 6 inches above its surface, clearing them of any negative energy that you intuit. Let them know that you are clearing them of any pain, hurt, judgment, and any other negative energy that may be held in their body so that they are totally clear. Have them continue to release any negativity with their out-breath.

6. While their eyes are still open so that they see the crystals, surround their body with four, six, or eight alternating green malachite and light green crystals. As you lay them down, say to the person, "These crystals will bring you the life force and healing of Mother Nature. "As I lay these crystals around you, let this nurturing and accepting energy enter into your body."

7. Ask them to now close their eyes and imagine that they see this green vitality of nature enter their body as beautiful, gentle, clear, green light until it fills their entire body. Guide them to imagine that so much light fills their body that it spills outward to surround them in an orb of green light that extends outward as far as they can see.

8. Have them continue breathing in and out of their heart energy center.

9. Now, place an amethyst or other violet crystal above their head with its tip pointing outward from their crown. Circle your clear crystal three times clockwise over the top of their head and around the amethyst or violet crystal to help open their crown energy center. Say to them, "I have placed a beautiful amethyst (or other violet) crystal over the top of your head. Imagine that the top of your head flowers open and a violet ray of healing, spiritual energy flows into the top of your head to fill your body with its light of wisdom and infinite peace." Use your clear crystal in your right hand to trace a line from the top of their head down through their body and out of the

(Continued on next page)

bottoms of their feet into the earth. See them as filled with violet light.

10. As you bring the violet light down into their body, ask them to feel as if their breath flows in through the top of their head with their in-breath and out from their heart center with the out-breath. Following this, ask them to feel as if their in-breath enters in through their heart center and out through the top of their head. Ask them to continue this breathing pattern, in through the head and out through the heart, then in through the heart and out through the head. Do this for at least three minutes, balancing the energy of the crown with the open heart.

11. After three minutes, ask the person, "What is something negative that you think about yourself? Just say the first thing that comes into your head." If they cannot think of anything (or are unwilling to reveal this thought to you), ask them, "If you had something negative about yourself, what would it be?" *Let them know that nothing they say will shock you or make you think less of them, and what they say to you is completely confidential.* As they reveal this, have them breathe in and out of their heart energy center.

12. Now ask them "How do you feel about this?" Then ask "Where do you feel this in your body?" If they can't identify a feeling or where it affects their body, ask them, "If you could imagine a feeling, what would it be? If you could imagine it being in your body, where would it be?"

13. Have them continue to breathe in and out of their heart energy center. Then ask them, "Are you willing to release this negative thought?" If they say that they cannot or will not, ask them, "What thoughts do you have about not releasing this negative thought about yourself?" After they have relayed these thoughts, then say, "I am going to help you release these negative thoughts." Have them continue to breathe in and out of their heart center.

14. Use your clear quartz crystal to "hook" or "scoop up" these thoughts, lift them out of the heart center, and send them into Mother Earth as

you touch the tip of the crystal to the ground. Let them know what you are doing as you do it and have them continue to breathe in and out of their heart center.

15. When you are through, ask them if they are now willing to replace this thought or belief about themselves with a positive thought about themselves. If they could think of a positive thought about themselves, what would it be? If they are not willing to think of a positive thought, tell them to just imagine a positive thought. Then continue to repeat this positive thought as you use your clear quartz crystal to send the thought into their heart center, letting them know you are doing this. Ask them to visualize and concentrate on this positive thought entering their heart center, letting it enter with every in-breath, and relaxing with the out-breath. Continue sending the positive thought into their heart center for at least three minutes.

16. Once you are through, have them now focus on their heart center as they continue to breathe in and out of it. After three minutes of heart breathing, let them know the session is ending and that you are going to remove the crystals as they continue their heart breathing.

17. Remove the crystals in the opposite order in which you placed them, leaving the pink rose quartz, pink tourmaline, or other pink crystal last. Then have them open their eyes.

18. Ask the person you are working with to remember the positive thought that they chose and to repeat it throughout their daily life until your next session. Hand them the rose quartz, pink tourmaline, other pink crystal, an amethyst, or clear quartz crystal to keep with them, telling them that every time they feel it or see it, it will remind them to silently repeat the positive thought or belief as a positive affirmation.

19. Clear your crystals after the session and clear yourself. Do not clear the person you are working with so that they retain what they experienced during your session.

Very rarely will one session completely alleviate someone's depression, because usually there are quite a few negative beliefs or thoughts that a depressive person will have. Usually, these thought patterns are mutually supportive, which makes it even more difficult to positively transform them. It is best to have the person come back for a series of sessions, each session working with another belief or negative thought. Do not be surprised if you find yourself working with the same negative thought pattern more than once. You can ask the person to bring the crystal that you gave them back to each session to add the new thought pattern you worked with in each session, so that, eventually, the crystal will be programmed with all the positive thoughts that you have unearthed during the sessions.

I AM THE EMBODIMENT OF BEAUTY AND PERFECTION.

SUICIDE

Talking about or having feelings of suicide always needs to be taken seriously, even if someone frames it as "just joking" or that they're not being serious. When faced with someone with suicidal ideation, the first thing to do is ask the person if they have an actual plan. If they do, they are serious. Talk to them and don't be afraid that asking them about suicidal thoughts will push them into it. In fact, it may help them to talk to someone about it. Ask them things like, "Do you feel like giving up or hurting yourself? Have you ever tried to hurt yourself before, or have you ever thought about suicide before?"

If the person you are working with is suicidal, you should either call the suicide prevention line, seek a medical professional, call 911, or if is safe, take the person to the emergency room. Determine if they have overdosed on drugs or alcohol. You should also contact a family member

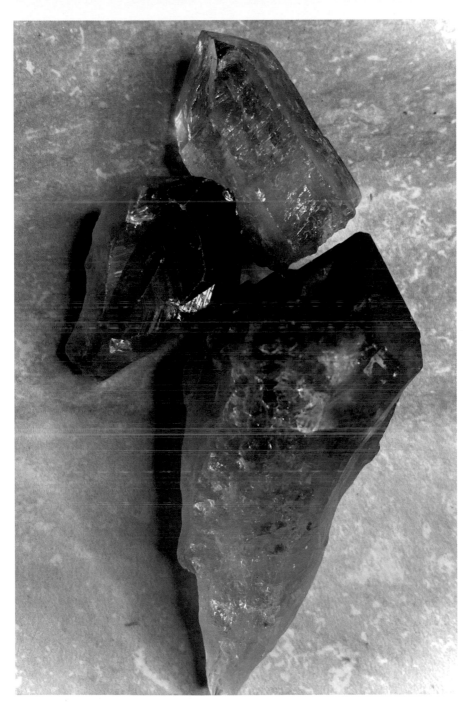

Dark Brazilian and Light Mexican Amethyst Crystals

or trusted friend who can help. If someone is truly suicidal, you should not leave them alone until someone arrives who can help them.

You can't always tell if someone is truly considering suicide, but here are some signs:

- Talking about suicide, saying things like "I should never have been born" or "I wish I were dead."
- Having a plan or gathering the means to end their life like stock-piling pills or buying a weapon.
- Wanting to be left alone and withdrawing from all social contact.
- Changing their normal routine, sleeping, or eating patterns.
- Having extreme mood swings or doing risky or self-destructive things.
- Giving away their belongings, getting their affairs in order, or saying goodbye to people.
- Being preoccupied with death or violence.

Finally, it is important to avoid worrying about intervening. When you are with someone who is suicidal, it is easy to think that your intervention might make things worse, but nonetheless, the best thing you can do is take action. Above all, *don't try to handle it alone.*

WHEN FACED WITH SUICIDE, ALWAYS INTERVENE.

The Ultimate Guide to Emotional Healing with Crystals & Stones

SECTION SEVEN
CRYSTAL AND STONE HEALING FOR CORE CHILDHOOD WOUNDING

Deep, core wounds can occur when a parent or important early caregiver with the same core wound withholds love from the child and passes their own wounding to you. Whether from this generational wounding or not, these core wounds stem from traumatic experiences in early childhood in which love and acceptance were withdrawn or nonexistent. These experiences form the basis for deep, lifelong, emotional pain. If you find that the emotional turmoil has been lifelong rather than from a more recent occurrence, that it persists no matter what you do, it is highly likely that it is core wounding in response to early childhood trauma. As was described earlier, this deep wounding is suppressed emotional pain resulting from a significant event. From this original pain, a negative belief system was created by the child about others and themselves. This, then, leads the child to compensate with certain behaviors and feelings that become a way to avoid experiencing the traumatic pain of the original wound. These compensating beliefs, emotions, and behaviors carry on into adulthood. Besides being painful, they limit the ability to form healthy relationships, to live with full and satisfying self-expression, and ultimately to give and receive love.

There are certain feelings and behaviors that result from core wounding that are traditional and that you will face in your emotional healing work with yourself and with others. You will need to be able to

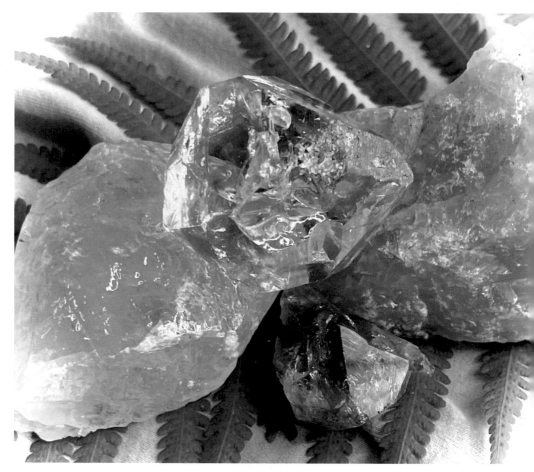

Green Calcite, Herkimer Diamond, Rose Quartz, and Amethyst

recognize these traditional core wounds and then discern and reveal the emotional layers that serve to protect from the re-experiencing of the core wound. Then you will need to heal each emotional layer to finally heal the core wound itself.

This is not something you can do in one or a few sessions. You will need to have many, with each session designed to work with one layer of healing. Once it is resolved, then you can move on to the underlying layer of emotional pain until you reach the original wound. This original wound is most likely to be the most difficult one to work with since it is so deeply painful and so fundamental to the core of the person.

How you can work with emotional layering has already been explained. Many of the crystal healing techniques that will work with both the emotional layers as well as the core emotional wound have already been described, as well. A crystal technique for healing shame, for example, has already been given to you. It will work for more recent or superficial emotional pain as well as for the deeper shame that results from early childhood ridicule or humiliation by the parent or primary caretaker. The technique of healing shame is not different for superficial or deep wounding. What is different is how to discover its source since, in deep wounding, the source of the shame is so deeply defended. So, not only will you have to work to heal the shame, but you will also have to work to heal the defense.

The Five Steps for Healing Core Emotional Wounds

There are five steps to take when you are working to heal the emotional effects of core wounding. Below is an explanation of each step along with an accompanying crystal and stone layout that will help assist the process.

All of the crystal and stone layouts start with the person lying on his or her back with their head straight, legs uncrossed, and their hands down at their sides with palms upward in receptive position. Their eyes should be closed. Then lay the crystals and stones down on and around the body as instructed, describing to the person each crystal and where you are placing it and why. Have the person breathe with slow, steady, deep breaths as if they are flowing in and out of the heart energy center in the middle of their chest unless instructed otherwise.

Here are the steps and crystal layouts:

STEP ONE: HEAL AND EXPLORE CURRENT EMOTIONAL PAIN

Ask the person to explain the emotional pain that is being felt. Instead of avoiding feeling the emotional pain, help them experience it as completely as they can, including how it makes them feel about themself and where it is stored in the body. (It is always stored in the body somewhere.) Do the crystal and stone healing work to help heal these first layers of emotional pain.

BASIC CRYSTAL AND STONE LAYOUT TO HEAL CURRENT EMOTIONS

You can use this layout for all emotional work. If the emotional patterns are those that have already been explained earlier, use those crystal healing patterns.

1. Place a rose quartz, pink tourmaline, or pink crystal on their heart center. Place four green crystals around it, one above, one below, and one on each side. This will help access the emotions and open the heart center.
2. Surround their body about 6 to 8 inches from its surface with black tourmaline or black crystals to bring them a sense of protection.
3. Place a smoky quartz below their feet, tip facing down, outside of the black crystal circle. This will allow the negative feelings to be channeled into Mother Earth, where they are positively transmuted.
4. Place an amethyst or violet crystal over the top of their head, its tip pointing upward, outside of the black crystal circle. This will help bring healing and higher wisdom.
5. Place a rose quartz or pink crystal in each upward-facing palm.

The Ultimate Guide to Emotional Healing with Crystals & Stones

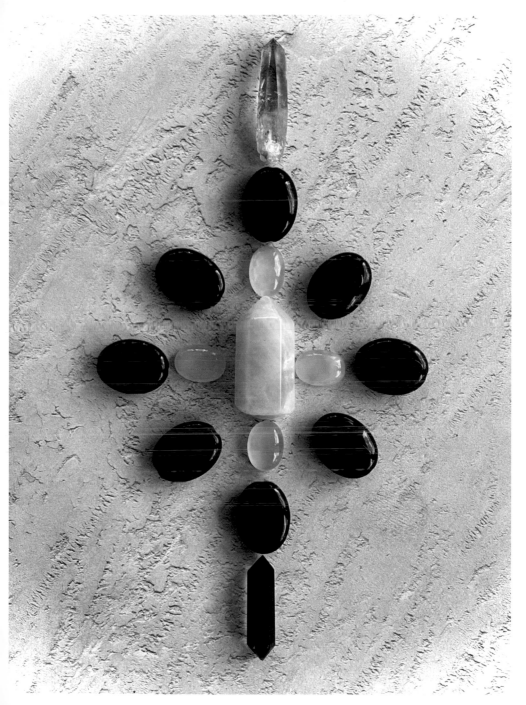

Crystal Layout to Heal Current Emotional Upset

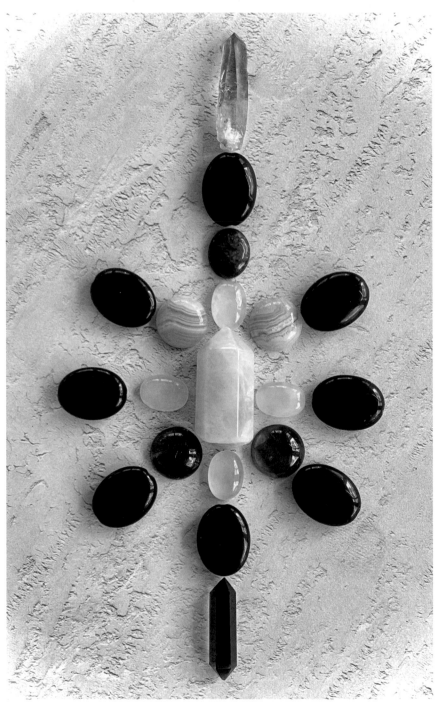

Crystal Layout for Exploring Avoidance Behaviors

STEP TWO: EXPLORE BEHAVIORS THAT HELP AVOID THE EXPERIENCE OF PAINFUL FEELINGS

Ask the person if they are aware of anything they do to keep them from having to experience whatever it is they don't want to feel. What do they do to keep the painful feelings away? If they can't find any such behavior, ask them to *imagine* feeling the painful emotion, and then *imagine* what they would do to avoid feeling it. (Asking someone to imagine something will trick the mind by suggesting that what is imagined is "not real," even though it is the truth. This way, it is not threatening.) Ask the person to imagine not doing the avoidant behavior. Ask them how they feel now when they imagine not doing this behavior. Ask them if they would be willing to release the behavior.

CRYSTAL LAYOUT FOR EXPLORING AVOIDANCE BEHAVIORS

1. Continue using the crystal and stone layout above.
2. Place a royal blue lapis, azurite, or other royal blue crystal or stone on their third eye energy center in the middle of their forehead. This will help bring insight and assist imagination.
3. Place two blue lace agates on their chest, each one between the nipple and the shoulder. This will help their breathing remain steady and calm rather than becoming rapid. It will also help them relax their chest when they imagine not doing a defensive behavior.
4. Place an amethyst slightly beneath the back above each hip. Point the tips downward if they are terminated. This will help relax the back as they imagine not doing the avoidant behavior.

STEP THREE: REVEAL LAYERS OF UNDERLYING FEELINGS UNTIL THE CORE WOUND IS REVEALED

Once you have worked to transform or reduce the pain of the original set of painful emotions, and after you have helped relax the associated behaviors, encourage the person to dig deeper. Help them discover the

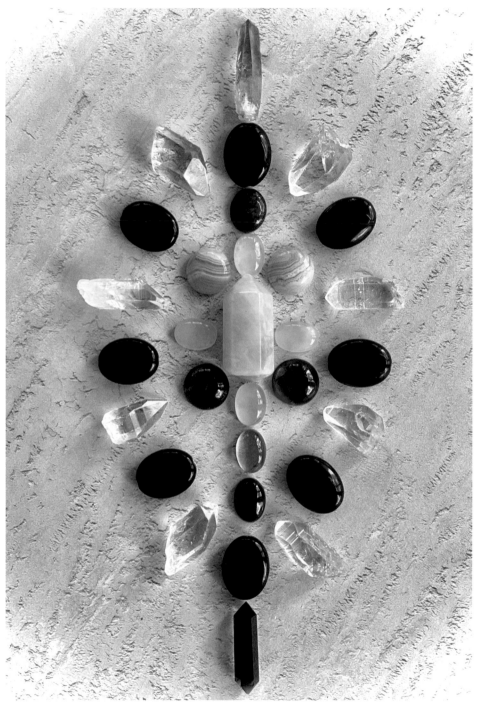

Crystal Layout to Release Underlying Feelings and Uncover Core Wounds

underlying painful or traumatic feelings that support the original, more outward ones. After letting the person know that there are likely deeper feelings that are buried in their subconsciousness, ask them if they would be willing to explore and relieve these. (Asking the person lets them know that you don't want to *do* something to them, that you merely want *to assist* in an exploratory process. This lets them know that you respect their ability to take charge of their own healing process. This empowers the person rather than making them reliant on you.) Encourage the unmaking of these underlying feelings by asking the person being healed, "Do you remember feeling this way before? When do you feel this way? Can you think of any experiences in the past that contributed to this feeling?" As you discover these deeper feelings then work to release them in the same way that you have done before, ask them if they would be willing to release them. If so, have them visualize the feelings being released into the earth, where they are positively transmuted. Work layer by layer, continuing to uncover underlying feelings and release them into the earth. This process may take several sessions.

CRYSTAL LAYOUT TO RELEASE UNDERLYING FEELINGS AND UNCOVER CORE WOUNDS

1. Use the same layout as step one.
2. Use a clear, natural quartz crystal to "lift" the painful feelings from their heart center and then send them into the earth, where they are positively transformed. Do this as they are describing and experiencing their feelings. Describe what you are doing with your crystal as you are doing it so that it is a mutually participatory process. As you do this, you can have them imagine that their feelings are being sent into the earth.

(Continued on next page)

3. To help them release painful feelings, have them imagine the feelings flowing into a round balloon that then slowly rises to fly away into the heavens, removing their painful feelings as it does so. (This visualization was described in more detail earlier in this book.)

4. When the core wound is revealed, place a bright yellow jade or citrine on their belly button and a garnet or red crystal beneath their tailbone, letting them know that these crystals will bring them strength to withstand any feeling, that nothing will be too intense for them to handle that they may find revealed.

5. Add a clear quartz crystal in between each of the black tourmaline or other black crystals around their body to strengthen the protective shield. Inform the person that you are doing this, letting them know that this will make them even stronger, and it will protect them from fright or anything terrible happening to them.

STEP FOUR: UNCOVER DECISIONS THAT WERE MADE WHEN EXPERIENCING THE ORIGINAL TRAUMATIC EVENT

Once the original emotional wound is uncovered, and the person feels a sense of strength and protection, use guided visualization to help them re-experience the traumatic episode as if they were a child. (This is a vitally important and incredibly sensitive part of the healing process and should be done carefully.) Ask them how they are feeling as they experience this event. Let them know that it is okay for them to show feelings that they were not allowed to show at that time. Let them know that it is safe to experience them now with you. Also let them now that you will not think any less of them, that they are totally safe in this space with you. It is important that you allow them to totally experience these feelings rather than immediately trying to get rid of them or repressing them as they did in childhood. Let yourself experience these feelings with the person, remaining open and empathetic. Rather than getting lost in them, however, as you feel them, take a deep breath inward, and then release it along with the feelings and imagine them flowing into the earth.

Once the person has thoroughly experienced these feelings, ask them how they feel about themselves. It is helpful to guide them by asking them this way: "What are you thinking about yourself right now as you are in this situation?" Then, "If you could decide one thing about yourself right now, what would it be?" "Do you feel as if you have done something wrong? What is it?" Then, "Do you feel like a bad person? If so, describe why you are bad." Then ask, "What have you decided about other people?" "Have you made any decisions about how you have to be around people to avoid experiencing this trauma again?"

As they reveal each negative feeling about themselves and each decision they have made, ask if they would be willing to release it and replace it with one more positive. Then, as they repeat each decision and negative feeling about themselves, use visualization and your crystal to assist the releasing process. With each thought that you release, have them repeat, out loud or silently, "I am good. I am okay just as I am. It is safe to be myself." You can say these words to them yourself and have them repeat them after you. To end the session, after you have removed the crystals, recap the decisions you heard them make about themselves and other people. Ask if they can see how they still use these in their life today.

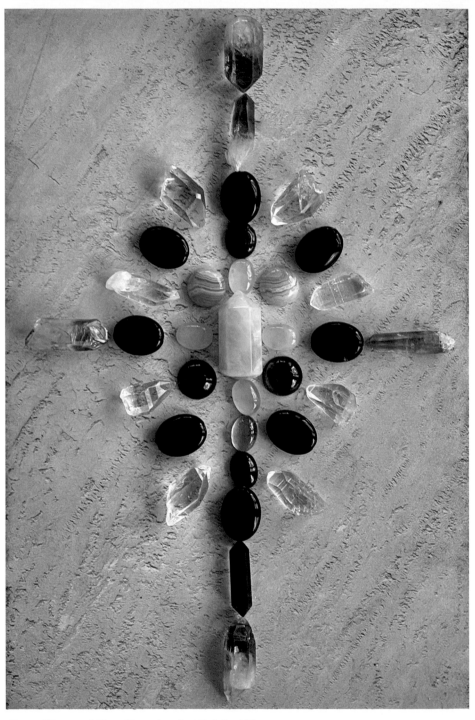

Crystal Layout When Experiencing Original Trauma

CRYSTAL LAYOUT WHEN EXPERIENCING THE ORIGINAL TRAUMA

1. Use the crystal and stone layout from the third step.
2. Replace the rose quartz in each hand with clear quartz crystals. If they are single terminated, point the tips up toward the arms. Tell the person being healed that these crystals will help bring power to them.
3. Add four more amethysts around the body about 6 inches outward from the crystals that already surround the body. Point their tips inward. Place one above the head, one on each side of the body, and another below the feet. Use your clear crystal to imagine a violet light connecting each amethyst crystal. Let the person being healed imagine that these crystals will bring total healing energy from the highest heavens.
4. Use your clear crystal to help release all negative feelings and decisions as they are revealed.

STEP FIVE: REFRAMING THE CORE WOUNDING EVENT

Using guided visualization, revisit that original wounding experience and see it from the eyes of the adult they are now. Reframe it so that the person being healed no longer blames themselves, accepting that they are not at fault for how the other person (usually a parent or primary caretaker) acted, reacted, or felt. With this new understanding, help the person release the old feelings about themselves and accept a new, positive understanding.

For example, with the viewpoint and understanding of the adult that you are now, as you view your parent constantly yelling at you, maybe saying things like "I hate you" or "I wish you had never been born," you may now understand that they were totally overwhelmed, possibly raising their kids without help or without sufficient money. You may also

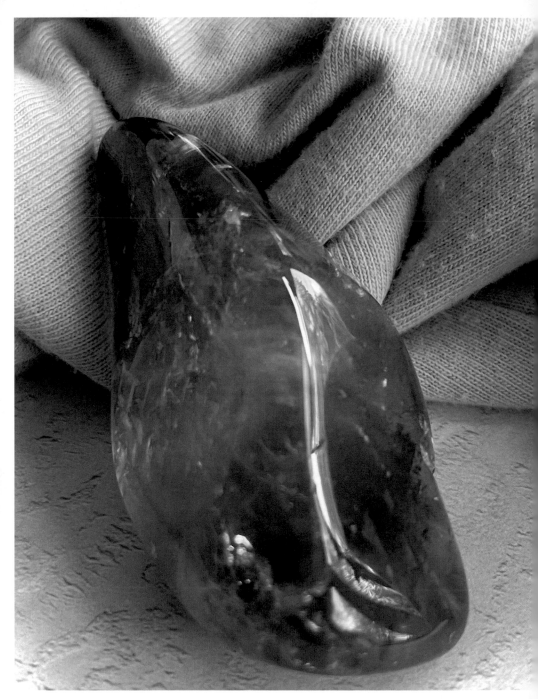

Soothing Amethyst Hand Crystal

see that they often suffered from debilitating migraine headaches. With the eyes of the adult that you are now, you can understand that they probably didn't really hate you. Instead, they were at their wits' end and just reacting in frustration and anger at their life in general. Seeing that with the vision and life understanding of an adult, you now realize that it didn't really have anything to do with you. Nor was it really a judgment of your worthiness. With the clearer understanding of the event and the unconscious negative self-decisions made, you will then be able to help transform the negative and limiting self-beliefs to those that are more positive.

CRYSTAL AND STONE LAYOUT FOR REFRAMING

You can use the same layout as the one in the fourth step. It is helpful to remind the person being healed which crystals and stone are being used, and as you lay them in place, describe what they are for. Have an amethyst crystal at the session that you can give to the person being healed at the end of the session, letting them know that this crystal has "recorded" the entire process of healing. As they carry this crystal with them, it will remind them of their new understanding and their healing. Again, since this is such a powerful process at this point, let the person know that they are totally safe, that you are involved in this process with them, that nothing they say will make you think less of them, that they are powerful, and that they are a good person. Continue using your clear crystal to assist the healing process, "lifting" out any negativity and sending it into the earth. Be sure to clear yourself, the person being healed, and all the crystals after the healing session.

(Bonus) STEP SIX: FORGIVENESS

The final step in this healing process is to forgive the parent or primary caretaker of any harm that they may have inadvertently or knowledgably caused you. This doesn't mean that you must condone or approve of what they did to forgive them. You can still disapprove of their actions and still offer forgiveness. When you forgive, it means that you will no longer carry the effects of the harm within you, that how they treated you will no longer determine your self-opinion or affect your actions in the world. This is the final freedom from all core wounding.

FORGIVENESS BRINGS FREEDOM.

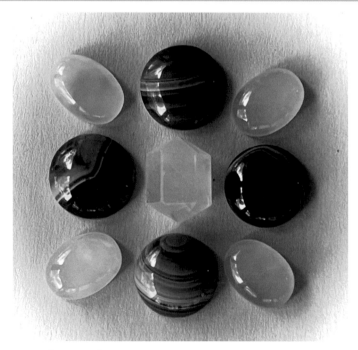

Crystal Layout for Forgiveness

CRYSTAL AND STONE LAYOUT FOR FORGIVENESS

You can use the crystal layout and forgiveness technique in the prior chapter. You can also use this one that is specific for core wounding:

1. Place a rose quartz, pink tourmaline, or pink crystal on your heart energy center. Surround it with four green crystals, one above, one on each side, and one below.

2. Hold a pink crystal in your right hand. If it is single terminated, point the tip outward toward your fingertips. This will help transmit or send the forgiveness energetically.

3. Hold a clear quartz single-terminated crystal in your left hand with its tip pointing in towards your arm.

4. Surround your body with four, six, or eight green crystals, preferably using green calcite or soft, light-green crystals.

5. Imagine the person to whom you want to offer forgiveness, seeing them clearly in your mind's eye. When you can visualize them clearly, point your right-hand pink crystal toward them and say the words, "I forgive you for all the ways you have intentionally or unintentionally harmed me." If you like, you can imagine a specific event, or specific incidents, and forgive the person with each one that you view in your mind's eye. Visualize the forgiving energy flowing from your heart energy center, down your right arm, and out of the pink crystal in your right hand.

6. At the same time, hold the clear quartz that you have in your right hand on your heart center in the middle of your chest. After each time you offer and send your forgiveness, take a gentle, deep breath, filling your lungs completely, and imagine that loving and forgiving energy fills your heart. Do this for at least three minutes or until you feel complete.

(Continued on next page)

7. Then repeat "I forgive myself for all the ways I may have intentionally or unintentionally harmed you." As you say this, use the same techniques with your pink and clear crystals. Do this for at least three minutes or until you feel complete.

8. Next, repeat the words "May you be happy and at peace." As you say this, point the crystals in both hands outward as if you are transmitting this blessing.

9. Continue doing this process or at least three minutes or until you feel complete. You can do this forgiveness process for as long as you like. There is no time limit.

Typical Core Emotional Wounds and Their Healing

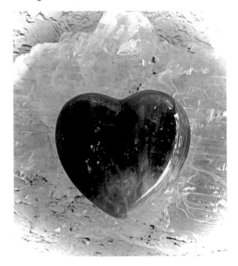

The following is a list of the typical emotional wounds and how they form. When you know what these typical wounds are, you can more easily spot emotional patterns and have some idea of how they formed. Then it will be easier for you to know the probable emotional layers and their genesis so you will be able to guide the revealing process more easily during the emotional healing work. Other crystals have been suggested that you can add to the layouts described above to accelerate the specific healings needed. Here are the typical core wounds:

SHAME WOUND

Origin of the Wound

The shame wound results from humiliation that you experienced as a child. You may have been ridiculed, laughed at, or embarrassed. Possibly you were exposed in a public way or were caught in a compromising situation that mortified you.

The Resulting Beliefs

As a result, you believe that you are a shameful person, that you deserve to be ridiculed, ignored, or treated with disgust. You believe yourself to be fundamentally unworthy of respect, that you are inherently "no good," or a "bad person."

The Compensating Behavior Adopted

You avoid all situations in which you may be ignored or treated with disgust. You may be shy, unable to look people in the eye, or otherwise withdraw from social interactions. You tend to unconsciously seek or attract people who treat or speak to you in a way that affirms your basic unworthiness. You may act out this belief in your own essential shamefulness by acting in dishonorable, reprehensible, or shameful ways. Or you do the opposite and act as if you believe yourself to be better than anyone else.

Healing

Learn to treat yourself with self-respect. Work to open the heart energy center and accept your own worthiness. Investigate the origins of your shameful feelings and use affirmations to affirm your sense of honor. Use a garnet to energize the root energy center at the base of the spine to develop a sense of belonging.

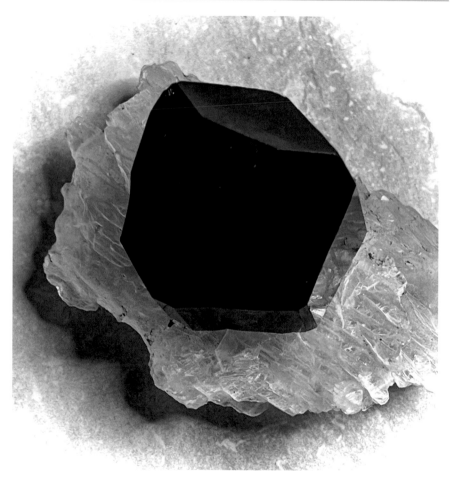

Natural Garnet Crystal on Selenite

The Ultimate Guide to Emotional Healing with Crystals & Stones

INADEQUACY WOUND

Origin of the Wound

The inadequacy or judgment wound originates from early negative judgment that is usually frequent and harsh. You may have been told that you never do anything right, or that you aren't good enough, that you don't live up to the parent's expectations, or they think you are a failure.

Resulting Beliefs

You tend to believe that you are a failure, that you will never be good enough or a success in anything you try. No one will like you since you are such a failure.

Compensating Behavior

You believe that you must be perfect in everything you do. You become a perfectionist and pressure yourself. You think there is only one right way, usually the way that is hard or impossible for you to achieve. To hide your sense of failure, either you withdraw from people or do the opposite and become a braggart, calling attention to everything that you do that you believe to be special.

Healing

It is healing to learn that you don't have to be perfect, nor does anyone else. Accept yourself as you are. Use a yellow crystal on your solar plexus to increase your sense of personal power.

> **I DO NOT HAVE TO BE PERFECT TO BE LOVED.**

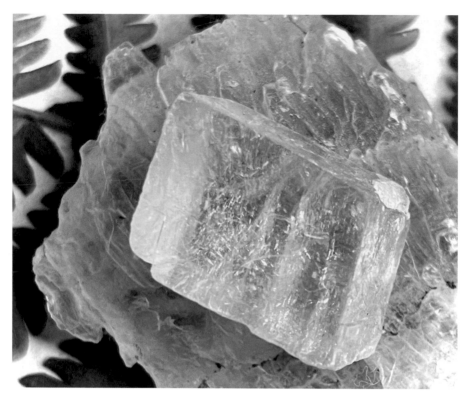

Yellow Fluorite

ANGER WOUND

Origin of the Wound

This wound has its origin from exposure to violence during early childhood. Or you were the recipient of violent behavior, constant uncontrolled angry explosions, or you were constantly yelled at. You may have been attacked or felt as if you were under attack.

Resulting Beliefs

If you are suffering from an anger or attack wound, you feel as if you are not safe in the world. You feel the need to hide behind a layer of physical, mental, or emotional protection. You believe that anger is not safe, whether you are the recipient of it or you are angry yourself. You are afraid to show your own anger. You are a "people pleaser," feeling that you always must be nice, calm, and understanding, accepting any of their behaviors as long as it isn't anger.

Compensating Behavior
You avoid any situation that may become violent. Because you are afraid of anger, you avoid it at almost all cost. You are also afraid of people's anger, so you either avoid doing anything that may make someone angry or you avoid angry people entirely. You are often afraid to assert yourself because you are afraid that someone may get mad at you. You often lack boundaries. You repress your own angry feelings. Or you may do the opposite and be unable to control your own expressions of anger. You may have constant temper tantrums and rage at people.

Healing
You need to learn to be comfortable with your own and others' anger. Work to reduce fear when in the presence of anger. If you constantly feel angry, you need to work with anger management, learning to control your anger and express yourself differently. Explore the source of your anger and learn to use your breath to create a calm mind. Long, deep breathing in and out of your heart center will help calm your anger as well as the use of a green crystal on the solar plexus power center.

I NO LONGER FEAR ANGER.

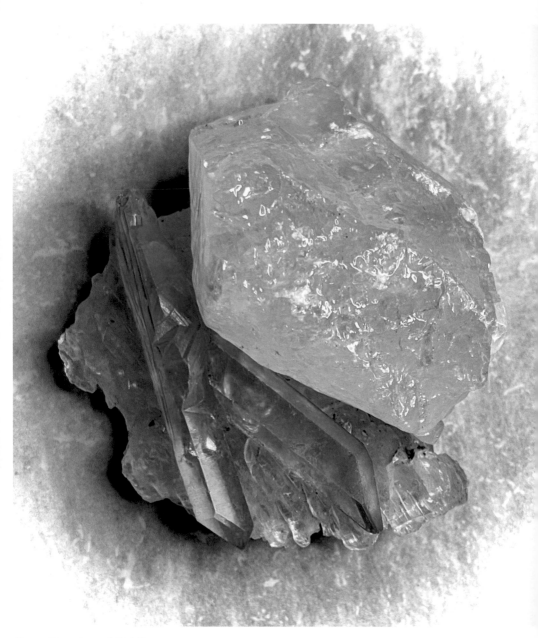

Green Quartz and Calcite

ABUSE WOUND

Origin of the Wound

The abuse wound originates with abuse. You may have suffered physical abuse in your childhood from parents, siblings, relatives, or other primary caretakers. You may have been raped or sexually assaulted, beaten, or constantly hit, locked in the dark, left without food, or seriously neglected, for example. The abuse wound is not reserved for physical abuse. You may have suffered from emotional or psychological abuse, as well.

Resulting Beliefs

People who suffered abuse in their early life may feel angry, shameful, or despairing. They can feel worthless with feelings of being "no good" or undeserving.

Compensating Behavior

Someone who has been abused is angry, whether they direct it outward or inward. Panic attacks and post-traumatic stress disorder often result from physical abuse. The victim of such abuse may develop symptoms of depression, anxiety, irritability, or become suicidal. This person may also do the opposite and direct their anger outward with various forms of aggression, become hyperactive, hypercritical, manipulative, controlling, possessive, or impulsive. They can become dismissive of others' feelings.

Healing

Learn how to have healthy boundaries. Learn to value yourself. Use extra tourmaline around your body for healthier boundaries, and an extra amethyst over your crown to relieve anxiety and depression and increase your spiritual connection.

I DESERVE LOVE AND TO BE SAFE FROM HARM.

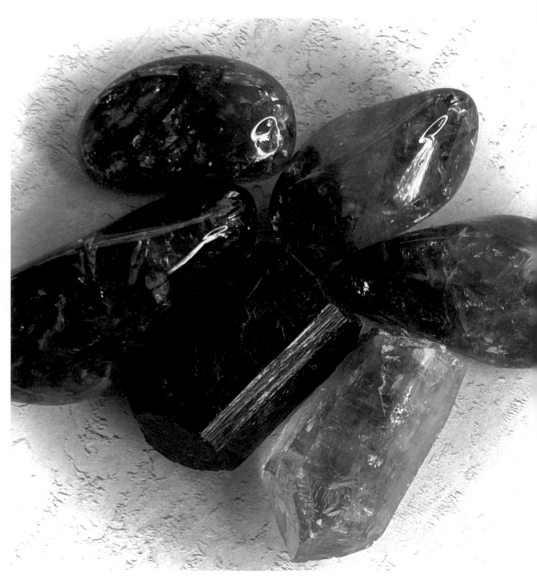

Amethyst and Black Tourmaline Crystals

DOMINATION WOUND
Origin of the Wound

This form of wounding results from being smothered, controlled, or otherwise violated in your early life. You may have had your personal space constantly violated. You felt that you were at the mercy of your parent or primary caretaker, rewarded only when you did what they wanted and punished if you didn't. They may have been an especially strict disciplinarian, been overprotective, treated you as a slave, or not allowed you to make your own life decisions, even when you were old enough to do so.

Resulting Beliefs

The domination wounding can create the belief that you have to be completely self-reliant so no one can control you again. Another belief is that you must be a rebel to get your way, that any compromise may result in being controlled. You may be afraid of intimacy, believing that if you get too close to people and let down your guard, they will cease respecting your boundaries.

Compensating Behavior

If you suffer a domination wound, you tend to keep yourself emotionally apart from people. You can be stubborn, not letting anyone telling you what to do. You may have trouble working as a team with others. You may have trouble being criticized or accepting others' opinions. These are all attempts to avoid any form of what may lead to domination by others. Or you may compensate by becoming a bully, overly dominating of others, not allowing the validity of other's opinions, and thinking that your opinion is the only right one.

Healing

Learn to open your heart and be close with people without dominating them. Learn to be comfortable with reliance on others. Learn to set up personal boundaries that also let people get close with you. Use tourmaline and garnet to help build a sense of protection and personal power.

I AM FREE TO BE MYSELF.

BETRAYAL WOUND

Origin of the Wound

This wound originates from being betrayed in some form by the important other person in your life, usually a parent or primary caretaker. This important person may have promised you something that they then failed to fulfill, or you may have trusted them to take care of you and they didn't. Similarly, you may have trusted someone to respect your needs, and they failed to do so.

Resulting Beliefs

When you suffer from a betrayal wound, you believe that people are basically untrustworthy, so you don't trust anyone. You feel unworthy of what others have, or of what life can offer, suffering from a lack of self-esteem. You may think, then, that since you are basically undeserving, you don't deserve happiness or success in life.

Compensating Behaviors

As a result of a betrayal wound, you may become rigid, having to control people. You need to have everything exactly as you want it. You may become intolerant and afraid or unable to be alone. This feeling of mistrust can also express itself as envy, feeling like you have missed out

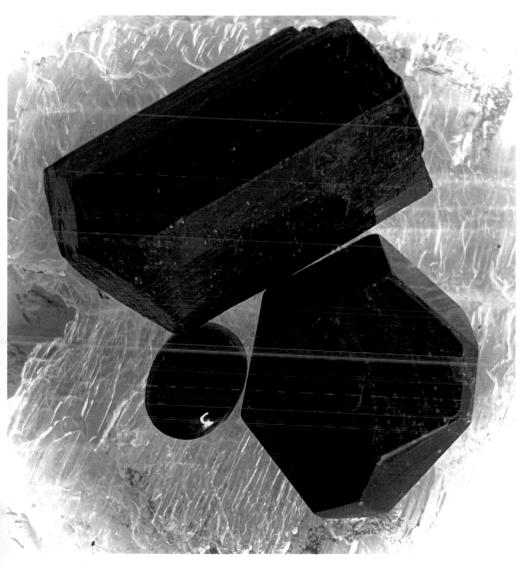

Garnet and Black Tourmaline

whenever someone has or does something that you want for yourself. You may have trouble maintaining relationships, either being hyper-aware of possible betrayal, or doing the opposite and ignoring signs of betrayal to stay in relationship.

Healing

Work to reduce your envy if you are envious. Learn to be tolerant of others. Open your heart to be able to trust yourself and others. Use more crystals and extra focus on the heart energy center.

I OPEN MY HEART TO TRUST.

REJECTION WOUND

Origin of the Wound

The origin of this core wound is disconnection or dismissal by your parents or your early caregivers. You were treated as if you were unimportant, or you were ignored completely.

Resulting Beliefs

When you suffer from the rejection wound, you believe that people aren't going to like you. You think of yourself as inadequate or lacking, or that something is fundamentally wrong with you. You believe that because you were rejected, you are not good enough for love, or that you're not attractive, too emotional, or that something in your being makes you unlovable.

Compensating Behaviors

To compensate for these beliefs, you reject others before they can reject you. You may choose people to be in relationship with you who are

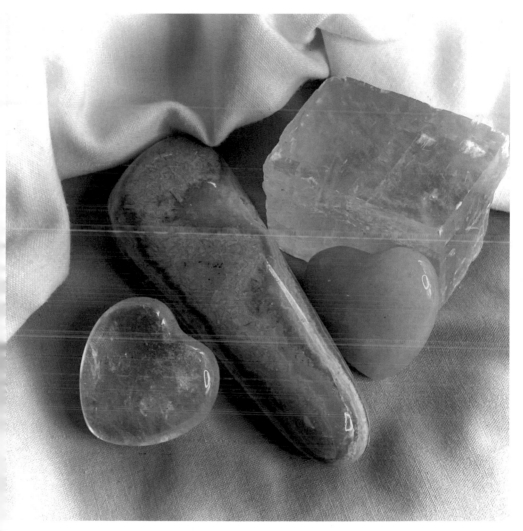

Clear Quartz, Rhodochrosite, Rose Quartz, and Pink Calcite Crystals

not interested, or you attract people who are trying to change you to be in a relationship with you. If you do find love and relationship, you will never be convinced that they really care for you, and if there are problems, you tend to flee rather than work it out. You project a perfect image and hide what you think are your flaws. If your rejection wound is severe, you don't think you even have a right to exist.

Healing

You have a right to exist. You are good enough and deserve love. Not everyone has to like you, and it is not a negative judgment of you if someone is not attracted to you. It is normal for people to feel attracted to others, or not. Open your heart and love yourself as you are. Use extra crystals on your heart center and over your crown for spiritual connection.

I AM IMPORTANT.

ABANDONMENT WOUND

Origin of the Wound

This core wound results from being physically, mentally, or emotionally abandoned by your parents or important caregivers in your early life. This abandonment may take many forms, among them, dismissing you, devaluing you, or not acknowledging you. It may also be caused when one of your parents has chosen not to be in your life or is absent, usually by the death of the parent or divorce.

Resulting Beliefs

As a result of this type of core wounding, you are afraid of being left again, especially in your important relationships. You doubt yourself and

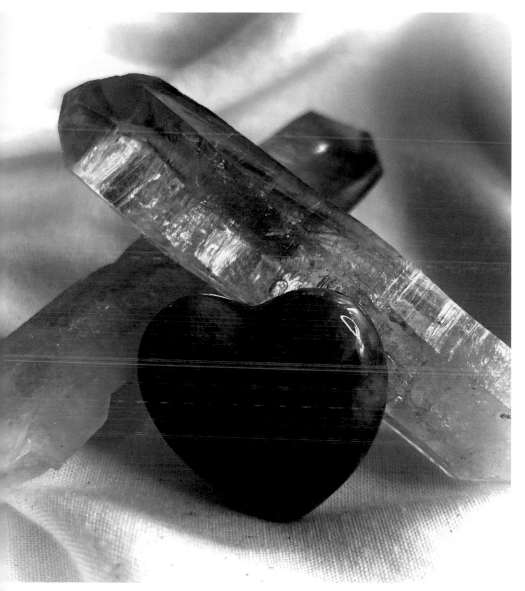

Amethyst

your place in the world. You tend to believe that you are worthless. You regard others as untrustworthy and think that others will always leave you.

Compensating Behaviors
Fearing abandonment yourself, you may hesitate to get into relationships or keep them on a "safe" or shallow level, so when you are abandoned again, it won't hurt as much. However, if you do allow someone to become close to you and feel threatened, you will tend to react with volatile anger, aggression, or other forms of emotionally reactive behavior. An opposite adaptive behavior is that you become codependent, clingy, or very needy in your relationships, always needing reassurance. You tend to be insecure, worrying about possible future disappointments or threatening losses in your life.

Healing
Learn that you have value just as you are, that you are worthy of love and caring. Open your heart center and transform your sadness. Release the expectation of being abandoned. Also use a yellow crystal on your navel point energy center to bring a sense of personal power and worthiness.

IT IS SAFE FOR ME TO BE IN RELATIONSHIP.

GUILT WOUND
Origin of the Wound
The guilt core wound, also resulting from early childhood trauma, may have developed if you were repeatedly made to feel guilty for the things you did. You may have been made to feel guilty if you asked for things and were made to feel as if you weren't deserving. You may have been

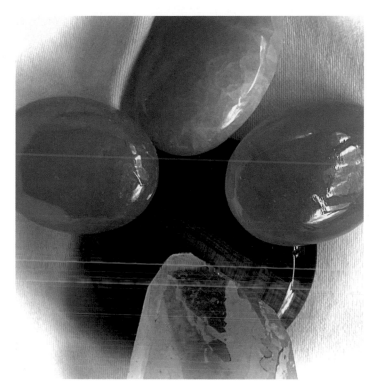

Gold Tiger Eye, Yellow Jade, and Citrine

punished using guilt for violating your family's moral beliefs or your family's cultural beliefs. You may have grown up in a family that used guilt as a punishment or a way to influence your behavior, or it was used to influence other people. Your parents or early caregivers may have blamed you for their own emotional problems. Or you may have hurt someone important and were never forgiven.

Resulting Beliefs
Because you were never forgiven, you treat others in an unforgiving manner. You believe that you are guilty of things of which you have no

control. You may tend to be judgmental of others or make others feel guilty.

Compensating Behaviors
One of the compensating behaviors is that you feel like you must take care of others. You have trouble setting personal boundaries and let people take advantage of you. You tend to be very critical of yourself, and then feel guilty because you can never live up the level of criticism. You tend to get defensive whenever criticized so that you won't feel guilty. You may blame yourself for things for which you were not responsible.

Healing
You need to learn to become more nurturing of yourself. It is also helpful to learn to distinguish what is and what is not your responsibility. You need to learn to forgive yourself. Use extra crystals on your heart center.

I NO LONGER HAVE TO DEFEND MYSELF.

ACCEPTANCE OR NOT-SEEN WOUND
Origin of the Wound
This core wound originates in early childhood, occurring if you were not seen and appreciated by your parents or significant others. You were likely not seen for who you were or you remained unheard. You may not have been allowed to express yourself, or your accomplishments were not acknowledged. You were treated as if you were invisible. Your parent may have treated you as their own confidante, so your needs were not heard. You didn't feel acknowledged for who you truly were as a human being.

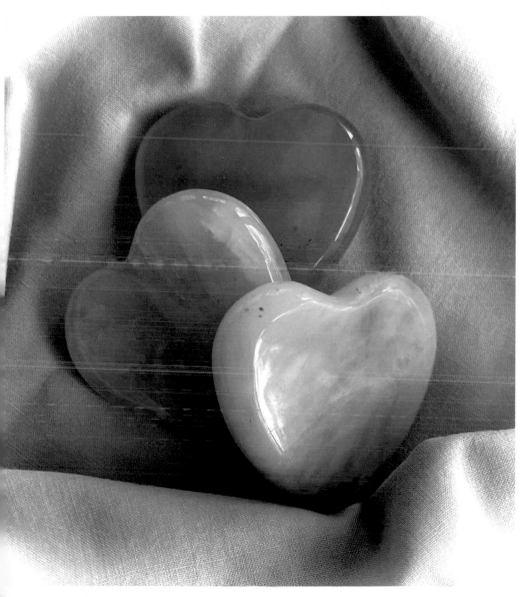

Green Jade and Rose Quartz Heart Crystals

Resulting Beliefs

You don't believe in your own value or worth as a human being, telling yourself that no one cares what you say or do. You believe that it is not safe to express your emotions. You believe that you should keep quiet about your beliefs and your viewpoint, and you should minimize what you do in life. You believe that it is not safe to be visible in life, that it is better to hide your authentic self.

Compensating Behaviors

You don't share your authentic self with others and withdraw socially. You don't see your own capability or don't believe in yourself. You are very careful to not "stand out," do anything better than other people so that you can have relationships with others. You may compensate by living like a foolish or crazy person. You stop having the energy to nurture your own talents and downgrade their importance to you and others. You tend to seek external approval from other people. You act out your feelings of aloneness and believe that you will always be misunderstood or rejected. Or you may exhibit behaviors of the other extreme, behaving in a tyrannical manner and rebelling against all forms of authority.

Healing

Learn to own and be comfortable with your own uniqueness, to cherish and value yourself. Do work to be able to accept yourself as you are and to realize your own value. Discover, acknowledge, and accept your own unique talents. Release those inner restraints that keep you from shining and standing out in the world. Appreciate yourself and learn to become emotionally vulnerable. Use a yellow citrine on your solar plexus to increase your sense of personal power and turquoise on your throat center for self-expression.

The Ultimate Guide to Emotional Healing with Crystals & Stones

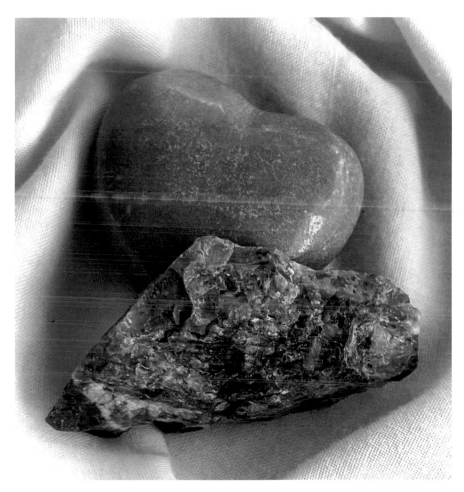

Turquoise and Yellow Jade

UNLOVABLE WOUND

Origin of the Wound

This core wound occurs when you were either rejected, dismissed, abandoned, or otherwise treated as if you were unlovable. Basically, you were not loved as a child. You may have been overlooked in favor of another child, or your parents were so busy that they failed to give you the loving attention that you deserved.

Resulting Beliefs

You believe that there is something wrong with you and that you don't deserve love or that you are basically unlovable. You view yourself as unworthy and have low self-esteem. You tend to be highly critical about yourself and may feel anxious and depressed. You may keep yourself isolated from others.

Compensating Behaviors

A usual compensating behavior is that you try to be perfect to win people's love and acceptance. You may become a people pleaser and constantly monitor others' moods to please them in order to be loved. As a result, you are constantly anxious and worried about others' feelings, more so than your own, believing yours are not as important. You may feel empty, numb, or apathetic to avoid feeling unlovable.

Healing

Open the heart energy center and flood yourself with love. Realize that the thoughts you have of being unlovable are only that—thoughts—and learn to change your thinking patterns of being unloved or unworthy. It is helpful to re-parent yourself, repeating the things to yourself that you wish you would have heard from your parents. Realize that how you were treated reflects your parents and not you. Use extra crystals on your heart center.

The Ultimate Guide to Emotional Healing with Crystals & Stones

Common Defensive Patterns

As you do your emotional healing work, you will likely have to work to deconstruct people's defensive patterns that they consciously or unconsciously use to protect themselves from experiencing their emotional pain from core wounding. These defensive patterns are powerful walls designed to keep others from recognizing their supposed personal flaws and imagined deficiencies as well as to mask their own emotional pain. These patterns, usually well established, first need to be recognized by you, brought to the attention of the person you are healing, and discussed before you can begin deconstructing them. Once you discover and discuss an emotional defensive wall, you must proceed with gentleness and great care. This can be a scary process for the person you are healing because it leaves them feeling vulnerable and exposed. This exposure that they fear risks having you abandon or think less of them and risks feeling the pain of the emotion that they are trying to suppress. They may even subconsciously or consciously fear their total physical, mental, or emotional destruction. As you do the six steps of the emotional healing process, part of it should be to uncover these defenses. A good way to do this, for example, is to say something like, "I notice that you seem angry even when you say that you are happy." Or "I notice that you are dismissive of me right now. Is there anyone else that you feel dismissive of?" If they deny that they are using a defensive method, you can work around that by asking them to *imagine* that they are feeling a way that they deny. For example, referring to the above example again, you can ask, "If you were angry, what would it be about?" or "Just imagine that you are angry for a moment. What does it feel like?" By asking them to

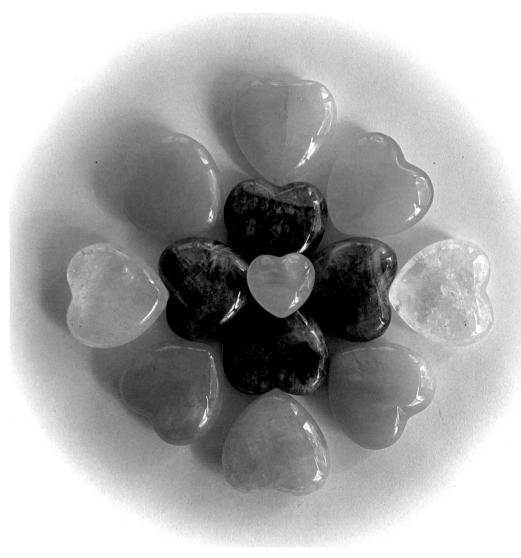

Crystal Mandala to Heal Core Wounding

imagine a defense, they don't have to risk immediately acknowledging it but can still talk about the emotional wound. Later, now that you have opened the topic, you can get more specific with them because now they are more comfortable talking about it.

The crystals that you have used for protection, personal power, opening the heart, connecting with spiritual higher awareness, and self-expression will all help with this process. If at any time if you feel that it will help with this deconstruction process, use your clear crystal to send power into the energy center that you think is more affected.

Here are the most typical defensive patterns that are in reaction to the core wounds that you will likely experience during your emotional healing sessions. Being able to recognize them will guide you in your work because it is only upon recognizing them that you have an opportunity to investigate and heal what lies beneath.

- **Denial**—They deny that the feeling exists, and believe that you are mistaken in your analysis.
- **Rationalization**—They justify their difficult, objectionable, or undesirable feelings with logical reasoning and explanation.
- **Repression**—They *unconsciously* keep the difficult or painful feelings from their conscious mind, so they don't have to feel them.
- **Suppression**—They *consciously* keep the painful feelings from their conscious mind.
- **Sublimation**—They convert unacceptable emotional reactions to those that are more acceptable. They may have an unhappy relationship with their child, so they channel their feelings into helping the elderly.
- **Displacement**—They transfer their painful feelings from one person to another. They may feel angry at their mother, perhaps, but yell at their wife instead.

- **Projection**—Denying painful or unacceptable feelings and instead ascribing them to someone else rather than themselves. Rather than experiencing their anxiety, they say that someone else is anxious.
- **Acting Out**—Rather than expressing a difficult feeling, they act in an extreme manner. Instead of saying "I hate you," they crash their car or throw a punch at someone.
- **Compensation**—They overachieve in one part of their life to compensate for other things that are wrong. They may feel like a failure, so they engage in risky behavior.
- **Reaction Formation**—They replace an unwanted feeling with its opposite. They may be feeling sad, but instead act happy.
- **Intellectualization**—They think about their painful feeling in a way that brings them emotional distance. They describe their feelings rather than experiencing them.

SELF-EXPRESSION WILL BRING ME HEALING.

The Ultimate Guide to Emotional Healing with Crystals & Stones

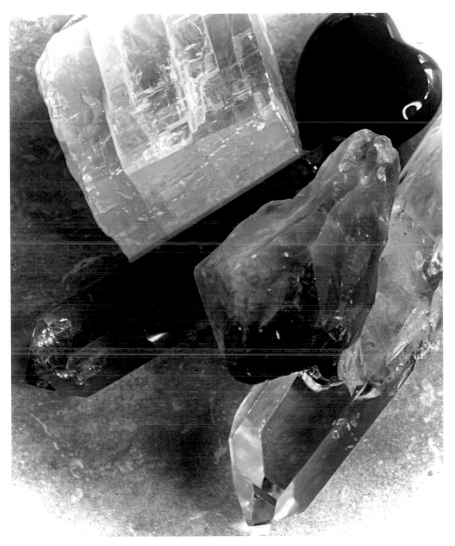

Red Jasper, Green Calcite, Amethyst, Yellow, and Smoky Quartz

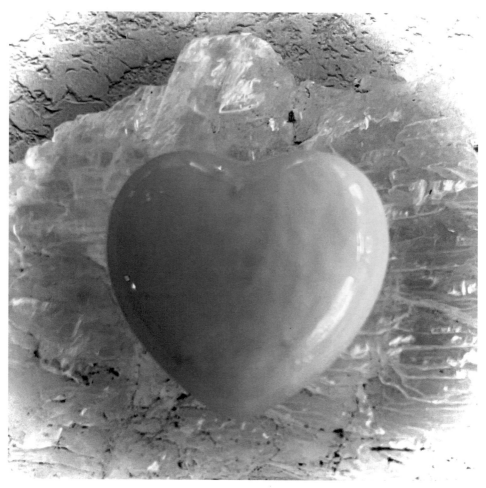

Green Jade Heart Crystal

CONCLUSION
WE ARE LARGER
THAN OUR FEELINGS

Whenever you are suffering emotional pain, it is easy to lose your perspective. When your feelings cause you suffering, your sense of self becomes consumed with your emotional state so much so that it seems like your feelings *are* your entire self. You *become* your feelings instead of merely *having* feelings. Battered with the pain and suffering of emotional trauma, you lose your anchoring to a secure sense of your own value, to your own sense of self.

No matter how much we hurt, or how large our feeling seems, it is helpful to know that we exist well beyond them. We are the larger field of awareness through which our feelings pass. In other words, our feelings come and go, yet who we are at our essence always remains the same. Our bodies, after all, are certainly different from when we were children. Our thoughts ceaselessly transform from one moment to the next, and our feelings are in constant movement. Yet the one who is aware, the one who witnesses, the essential beingness within which these transformations occur, always remains peaceful and unaffected.

When your feelings threaten to overwhelm you, instead of succumbing, with every breath, place your attention on this essential peacefulness, on your boundless, timeless, limitless peaceful self. Turn inward and immerse yourself in your sense of your own precious being. And you will be healed.

BE ONE WITH THE ONE.

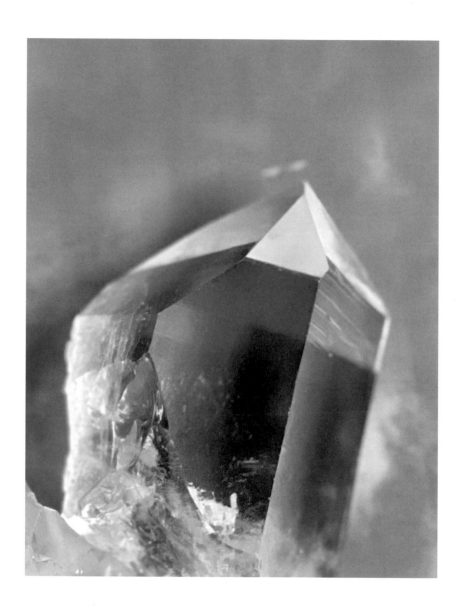

Healing Prayer

May golden
healing light
from the most high
heavenly spirit
pour through your crown's center
to fill your heart
with petals of wisdom
that flower
in the heart
of your Being.

May you be healed

Acknowledgments

Eternal thanks to my life partner, David Francisco, for always believing in me. And for his undying patience when the writing of this book turned me into such a hermit that he had to take up the household chores and forgo our normal, everyday life. If you had not been this patient and encouraging, this book would have been much harder to write.

Thanks also to my former husband, Paul Ramana Das Silbey, who encouraged me to start writing about my work with crystals in the early eighties and whose belief in me powered me onward.

Special thanks for my wonderful editor, Nicole Frail, of Skyhorse Publishing, whose meticulous editing helped shape this book to be as good as it could possibly be. Your trustworthy and precise editing "eye" is beyond wonderful. It is a joy, as always, to work with you.

To all my teachers, gurus, shamans, and medicine people who have passed along their knowledge, blessings, and empowerments; especially Sri Neem Karoli Baba, Sri Nisargadatta Maharaj, Siri Singh Sahab, Marcellus Bearheart Williams, H. H. Dalai Lama, H. H. Kalu Rimpoche, and all my psychology teachers at the University of California at Los Angeles (UCLA) and the California Institute of Integral Studies (CIIS) with whom I studied for ten years.

To my parents, who always encouraged me to follow my dreams and interests, and my sister, Sharon May, who listens, encourages, and inspires me. It is so special to have a sister who is also a friend.

And finally, to the formless, limitless, Sat Guru within. May we all listen and trust the inward guidance that we "hear."

Index

A

abandonment, 270–272

abuse, 263

acceptance, 274–277

affirmations, 171, 173

African malachite, green. *See* green African malachite

agate. *See* black agate; blue lace agate

allowing emotional change, 18

amber, 139–141

amethyst crystals, 22, 34, 36, 60–62, 141–142, 151, 231, 237, 240, 252, 264, 271, 283

anger, 175–179, 260–261

anxiety and anxiety disorders, 99, 179–183

apathy and emotional withdrawal, 189–194

aqua aura, 103, 113–116

avoidance behaviors, exploring, 244–245

azurite. *See* blue azurite

B

betrayal, 266–268

black agate, 77–79

black and gray crystals and stones

and boundary issues, 81–89

in the emotional healing kit, 72–81

and grounding, 90–91

black onyx, 75–77

black rutilated quartz, 98

black tourmaline, 72–75, 264, 267

blue azurite, 123–125

blue lace agate, 132–133

blue sapphire, 125–126

blue sodalite, 122–123

boundary issues, 81–89

breathing technique for a quiet mind, 20–21

C

calcite. *See* green calcite; pink calcite; white calcite; yellow calcite

centering yourself, 1

central cord of energy, 163

chakras. *See* energy centers, explanation of; higher energy centers, opening the

charoite. *See* violet charoite

childhood wounding. *See* core emotional wounds

circular patterns, 171

to reduce shyness and social anxiety, *216*

for relaxation, *153*

to release negative emotions, *44*

for releasing underlying feelings and uncovering core wounds, *246*

to relieve apathy, *191*

to remove or transform negative emotions, *47*

for a secure sense of self, *210*

for setting boundaries, *85*

for shielding from fear, *100*

for strength against fear, *202*

when experiencing original trauma, *250*

crystal techniques

for anger, 175–179

for anxiety, 181–183

for apathy and emotional withdrawal, 192–194

breathing for a quiet mind, 20–21

for current emotions, 242–244

for depression, 232–235

for developing a secure sense of self, 211–213

for emotional removal and transformation, 48–54

for experiencing original trauma, 251

for exploring avoidance behaviors, 245

for forgiveness, 185–188, 255–256

for grief, 197–199

for grounding, 91

meditation to be present-centered, 16

for obsessive compulsive anxiety disorder, 225–228

for opening higher energy centers, 24–27

for personal potency, 141

for reframing the core wounding event, 253

for relaxation, 154–155

for releasing underlying feelings and uncovering core wounds, 247–248

for sadness, 205–208

in setting boundaries, 86–89

for shame, 221–223

for shielding against fear, 101–102

for shyness and social anxiety, 215–218

for strength against fear, 201–203

for vitality, 138–139

crystals. *See also* specific crystals
preparation of, 4–7
storing and clearing of, 2–4
use of, without accompanying techniques, 33

current emotions, healing, 242–244

D

deep emotional wounding. *See* core emotional wounds

defensive behaviors, 52–53, 279–282
defensive pride, 221–223
depression, 229–236. *See also* sadness
developing self security, 211–213
disgust and contempt, 183–189
domination, 265–266
double terminated crystals, 6

E

early childhood events. *See* core
  emotional wounds
emotional abuse, 83–84
emotional healing kit
  amethyst crystals in, 60–62
  communication crystals and
    stones in the, 103–117
  heart crystals and stones in, 62–72
  insight crystals and stones in the,
    117–126
  list of crystals in the, 56–58
  protection and grounding crystals
    and stones in the, 72–91
  quartz crystals in, 58–60
  secondary crystals in the, 126–144
  solar crystals in the, 92–103
emotional healing sessions
  building trust with the, 145–150
  communication in, 105, 107–109
  crystal healing patterns, 157, 158,
    160, 163–171
  dealing with fear in, 99
  dealing with projection in, 82
  ending the, 54

establishing boundaries in, 86–87,
    88–89
  laying crystals and stones on the
    body, 157–162
  visualization and affirmation use
    in, 171–173
emotional projection, 40, 81–82
emotional removal and
  transformation, 45–46, 48–54
emotional withdrawal, 189–194
emotional wounds, core. *See* core
  emotional wounds
emotions, surface, 33–35
energy centers, explanation of,
  165–167. *See also* higher energy
  centers, opening the
envy and jealousy, 208–213
experiencing original trauma, 248–251
expressive crystals, 6

F

fear, 97–103, 200–203
fear of rejection, 214–218
fifth chakra, 165
first chakra, 165
fluorite. *See* purple fluorite; yellow
  fluorite
forgiveness, 254–256
fourth chakra, 165

G

garnet, 137–139, 258, 267
gold tiger eye, 98, 273

The Ultimate Guide to Emotional Healing with Crystals & Stones

green African malachite, 125, 130
green calcite, 34, 130–132, 240, 262, 283
green crystals and stones, 6, 7, 128–132, 231, 262, 275, 284
grief, 194–199
grounding, 1–2, 89–91
guilt, 272–274

H

heart center. *See also* fourth chakra
  crystals and stones for the, 56, 62–72
  and green crystals and stones, 128
  and method to be present-centered, 16
  stimulation of the, 6–7
Herkimer diamond crystals, 6, 56, 59, 60, 120, 159, 166, 240
higher energy centers, opening the, 21–27
howlite, white. *See* white howlite

I

identity and emotions, 51–52
imagined fears, 97–99
inadequacy, 259
insight crystals and stones, 57, 117–126
intention, 27–28
iolite. *See* purple iolite

J

jade. *See* yellow jade

jealousy, 208–213

L

lapis lazuli, 120–122
larimar, 103, 109, 110, 111, 116–117
lava, 98
layering of emotions, 35, 39–40
laying of crystals and stones on the body, 157–162
layout patterns. *See* crystal layout patterns
lepidolite, 135–136
listening, nonjudgmental and complete, 9–10

M

malachite. *See* green African malachite
manifestation and vibrational patterns, 11
meditation
  for anxiety relief, 181–183
  to be present-centered, 16
  and crystal visualization, 45–46
  for emotion removal and transformation, 48–54
  for observing the mind, 42–44
  preparing for, 1–2
mind/body connection, 29–32
mindfulness, 42–44
moon energy, 71–72
mother of pearl, 69–72

Notes

Notes

Notes

Notes

Notes

Notes

Notes

Also Available

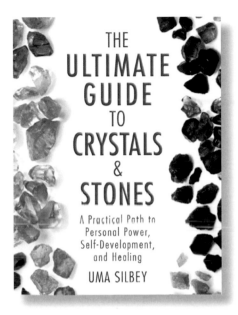

Ancient cultures referred to crystals as the veins of the earth, frozen liquid, and frozen light. Uma Silbey unlocks the secrets of these storehouses for earth's energy to reveal their remarkable effects on personal power, self-enhancement, and healing.

In this ultimate guide, she describes how you can channel the subtle forces within a crystal to empower your meditations, direct your thoughts, energize your body, and unleash a lifelong flow of creative and physical energy. From selecting the right crystal and "programming" it for your personal use to special techniques and exercises to heighten your abilities, Silbey guides you on the path to self-mastery. She provides information on:

- Different colors, shapes, and properties of quartz crystals and stones
- How to wear crystals and stones to take advantage of their protective powers
- How to heighten your crystal experience through visualization and meditation
- Insights into crystal gazing and crystal ball reading
- How crystals facilitate night dreaming and astral projection
- Crystal and stone techniques that can be used for healing physically, mentally, and emotionally
- And more!

Understanding the depth of our connection, crystals and all stones can assist us to become a conscious bridge between the macro and microworlds, help us to discern the patterns that create "reality," and, in so doing, facilitate healing, balance, and self-awareness.